THE NURSING PROCESS

Helen Yura, Ph.D., R.N., F.A.A.N.
Assistant Director
Division of Baccalaureate and Higher Degree Programs
National League for Nursing
New York, New York

Mary B. Walsh, M.S.N., R.N.
Associate Professor
Medical and Surgical Nursing
The Catholic University of America
Washington, D.C.

THE NURSING PROCESS

Assessing, Planning, Implementing, Evaluating

Third Edition

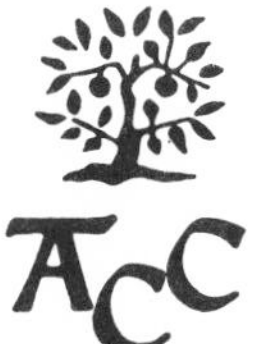

Appleton-Century-Crofts / New York

Helen Yura and Mary B. Walsh, The Nursing Process, Third Edition

A Publishing Division of Prentice-Hall, Inc.

79 80 81 82 / 10 9 8 7 6 5 4

Prentice-Hall International, Inc., London
Prentice-Hall of Australia, Pty. Ltd., Sydney
Prentice-Hall of India Private Limited, New Delhi
Prentice-Hall of Japan, Inc., Tokyo
Prentice-Hall of Southeast Asia (Pte.) Ltd., Singapore
Whitehall Books Ltd., Wellington, New Zealand

Library of Congress Catalog Number: 78-51077

Text design: Deborah Payne

PRINTED IN THE UNITED STATES OF AMERICA
0-8385-7032-1

This book
is dedicated to
our families

Contents

Preface

Analysis of the 1973 edition of *The Nursing Process* has revealed that certain areas of nursing have changed markedly, other areas have not changed at all, and a number of changes are in the "somewhat" range. We have been delighted with the responses of professional nurses to the nursing process publication and, even more, to the manner in which nurses have accepted the challenge to use the nursing process as a framework for nursing.

In this, the third edition, we present the developments in nursing as we perceive them. Our increased knowledge about the nursing process and reports about the changes it has wrought in nursing over these past five years are due in large part to the many persons with whom we have discussed the nursing process. Ideas about the use of the process, its relation to theoretical and conceptual development have come from persons in a variety of geographical areas. Enunciation of the process has increased greatly as is evidenced by the variety of activities and publications that receive the nursing process label, whether or not they accurately merit such a label. Application of the process to actual situations in nursing has varied, depending upon the abilities of the agents and the diligence, initiative, and creativity of the ones who are performing nursing. The number of publications with the nursing process label has increased by leaps and bounds during these five years.

In Chapter One, we have identified those events in nursing, significant to the nursing process, which have occurred since the second edition. The entire chapter has been revised and updated.

The theoretical frameworks presented in the 1973 edition continue to be appropriate. Additional content has been included in the areas of need theory and human problem solving theory. This content is fundamental to the performance of nursing and, although included by inference in the earlier text, it is identified specifically here to further identify the theoretical components of nursing.

The analysis of the nursing process components is not changed in format, nor has the essence of the process been revised in a major way. Areas of progress since the last edition have been added, mainly in the areas of nursing diagnosis and nursing evaluation.

A few new clinical situations have been suggested in Chapter Four. Feedback from readers suggested that there was limited revision needed in this section. Also, there are increased numbers of clinical situations being described in nursing periodicals where the nursing process is used as a framework for analysis and discussion.

A limited number of new directions are identified in Chapter Five. Despite the fact that many nursing education programs are using the nursing process as the curricular framework and despite the fact that the nursing service practitioners employ the nursing process in their activities, there is much more progress to be made in the use of the nursing process. The research potential identified in the 1973 edition has hardly been tapped, if one can use the nursing literature as an indication.

Appendix B has been retained in this third edition with expanded contents but in the same style as it appeared in the 1973 edition; a title has also been added. To our surprise, there has been little evidence that this material was seen, much less used in nursing. As emphasis on assessment continues to accelerate, and with continued concern for assistive devices for the nurse to use in assessment, perhaps the cues and clues provided in Appendix B will be of benefit to persons who are responsible for assessing clients' needs. Appendices C and D are new additions; they include the definitions and ABCD's of the nursing process phases, and an example of the application of the nursing process in reference to sensory deprivation.

Because of the marked increase in published data about the nursing process it is impossible to include an exhaustive bibliography. We have attempted to provide a variety of resources and settings where different interpretations and uses of the nursing process are explored and presented. The authors' intentions are to provide "springboards" of references from which the student and/or reader will be able to pursue individual interests and needs; therefore, extensive bibliographic additions have been made, and the format of the bibliography has been revised. The total readings are listed alphabetically rather than sectioned under different headings, as was done in the 1973 edition. The increased number of publications appropriate to the nursing process make it apparent that nurses are aware of the value of the nursing process; that this is where the emphasis on the nursing process is most evident is very heartening. There seems to be little doubt that an orderly systematic pursuit is the key to "good nursing."

Our continued gratitude is extended to all those practitioners of nursing who are making full use of the nursing process. We encourage your continued efforts. Special thanks is due to all those nurses who have shared with us their positive experiences and their difficulties in using the nursing process—this has been the means by which we have learned so much, and the essence of their experiences are the content of this, the third edition of *The Nursing Process.*

Special thanks is extended to Mary Bersin for typing the manuscript for this edition. Her meticulous typing, her dependability and her willingness are greatly appreciated.

H.Y.
M.W.

Preface to the Second Edition

The purpose of this book is to update data on the nursing process, data which we edited in 1967. The information presented in the seven papers of the 1967 Continuing Education Series at the Catholic University are incorporated in this book, which also includes pertinent data developed since the 1967 publication. A selective, though not exhaustive, review of the literature related to specific concepts and ideas about the nursing process which are of value to the baccalaureate nursing student are presented. Our views on the process are explained, and our philosophies and convictions about nursing are emphasized. The nursing setting is not limited to any one environment—home, clinic, hospital, or other agency—instead, we suggest uses of the nursing process in any setting in which there is a client, actual or potential. Several illustrations of the application of the nursing process will be presented; these can act as guides to those who use this book for teaching and learning purposes. We hope to stimulate ideas, activate thoughts and initiate actions.

This book is divided into five chapters: Chapter 1 briefly reviews the historic background and current ideas of the nursing process. Chapter 2 reviews some of the theories fundamental to and related to the nursing process. Chapter 3 analyzes and discusses phases of the process; chapter 4 suggests applications; and chapter 5 identifies future potentials in terms of study and research. A suggested reading list appears at the end of the book.

The word *client,* as used throughout this text, refers to an individual or family. It is our belief that nursing is practised in many settings, with a variety of consumers, few of whom possess a simple problem and all with some family, or at least significant person, concerned about them. Some consumers may have potential problems; the nurse must help the individual stay well. Some clients will have actual problems; the nurse's role is to help them to return to a state as normal for them as possible. The authors believe that the word *client* conveys this multifaceted concept of the consumer of nursing.

To facilitate readability, the pronoun *she* refers to the nurse; *he* refers to the client. No bias is intended in this use of pronouns; we trust our readers will understand and agree with us.

As the number of nurses who publish ideas and concepts about their profession increases, so does agreement about what nursing is and what the goals of nursing action are. Numerous nurses share the person-centered, goal-directed focus of their practice. In many instances, it is impossible to cite original ideas, for ours are molded and developed by the thoughts and ideas of many. Only a few specific ideas or particular contributions are cited in the text; this does not reflect the total number of nurses who have contributed. Many nurses will read their own ideas and convictions into those presented, since they undoubtedly developed these at the same time as the authors. We find it a positive indication that, in our discussions and in the literature, there is increasing evidence that nurses agree about our *raison d'etre*. This trend toward unified thinking among professional nurses reinforces the value of the nursing process as the core of nursing practice.

Were it not for the challenge and stimulation given by students with whom we have been associated for many years, this book would not have been possible. Our fellow faculty and our colleagues in nursing service stimulated ideas and encouraged us with their positive response to our development of the nursing process. We extend our appreciation to each of these persons and say: "Without you, this could not have been done!"

We are especially grateful to Ruth Lowe for her secretarial assistance, to Gloria Selitto who typed the manuscript, and to Ralph Selitto who drew the illustrations.

H.Y.
M.W.

THE NURSING PROCESS

Chapter One •

Historic Development of the Nursing Process

The nursing process is the core and essence of nursing; it is central to all nursing actions, applicable in any setting, within any frame of reference, any concept, theory, or philosophy. It is flexible and adaptable, adjustable to a number of variables, yet sufficiently structured so as to provide a base from which all systematic nursing actions can proceed. Phases, or steps, in the nursing process are identifiable. They can be examined, analyzed, and pursued deliberately by nurses as they provide care for clients. Although the exact labels identifying the phases of the nursing process may differ among groups of nurses and from one geographic area to another, there is a common theme underlying the process: it is organized, systematic, and deliberate.

Historic Events

Some reflection on certain historic events will be of benefit when considering the nursing process. Exact time periods are neither distinct nor precise, but the progress and developments that had a major impact on nursing can be grouped as follows:

1. Events preceding World War II
2. Events during World War II
3. Events following World War II
   a. During the 1940s and 1950s (1945–59)
   b. During the 1960s and 1970s (1960–78)

Events Preceding World War II

In the days of the early Christians, the practice of nursing was based on unselfishness and love of neighbor; there was concern for meeting the needs of each sick person. The actions of those who practiced nursing were directed toward helping the sick person get well so that he or she could lead a healthier and happier life. Persons who practiced nursing received little formal education. Most nursing behavior was learned by means of the apprenticeship system; the person who wanted to become a nurse accompanied an experienced practitioner, a role model, whose behavior was copied or imitated. Much nursing action depended on the judgments of experienced practitioners.

A history of people who lived during the Middle Ages reports that many persons cared for the sick; these persons responded, through their concern for people, to the social forces of the time to meet the basic human needs of the sick. During the last two centuries of the medieval period, many changes in national, political, and social structures occurred, all associated with the unrest and turmoil that necessarily accompany major change.[1]

As social forces and political structures changed, so did the practice of nursing; history records many phases with both high and low points through which nursing proceeded and survived. It was not until the days of Florence Nightingale (1820–1910) that nursing began to achieve some structure, some effort toward deliberate actions. In today's language, Florence Nightingale would have been called a *militant.* There was little establishment with which to disagree, yet she questioned traditions and customs that had been accepted for many years. She designed her own rules, and ran a very "tight ship" to achieve what she judged necessary to provide the best care for patients. Despite her maverick nature, she was farsighted and set admirable goals, establishing some firm foundations on which nursing continues to rest today. She emphasized knowledge, suggesting that the preparation needed by the staff nurse is different from that needed by a supervisor or an administrator. She was also concerned about just remuneration for nurses, although the 12-hour work day, the 7-day work week, and the 5-cent raise after a 6-month probationary period cannot compare with the work demands and pay of the mid-twentieth century. Regretfully, Florence Nightingale did not think kindly of male nurses, nor did she emphasize or even speak of the nursing process. Nevertheless, she deserves her title as the founder of modern nursing, having placed nursing on a respected and respectable level.[2]

During the years between Florence Nightingale's efforts and the beginning of World War II, there was little progress in nursing. These years can be called *the era of maintenance,* or *the era of little or no change.* World War I and the economic depression were among the reasons for this time of complacency in nursing. Other professions, as well as nursing, experienced similar lags in progress and merely maintained their status quo.

Events During World War II

World War II was a propelling force behind many changes in the world. The need for technology increased during this era. The health professions, especially nursing, felt the impact of this technologic change. War casualties increased the need for physicians and nurses; the pressures of war and feelings of patriotism created different ways to cope with human needs; the relatively uncomplicated triad of *doctor–nurse–client* gave way to a multidimensional health team, the dimensions of which have continued to grow and expand.

The contributions of medical corpsmen during the war set the pattern for auxiliary personnel in the health professions. As knowledge grew and accumulated rapidly, it became apparent that more persons were needed to cope with the consequent challenges. Advances in clinical medicine, such as early ambulation; changes and advances in the treatment of burns; and the discovery of new drugs, especially antibiotics, were forerunners of the changes that occurred in nursing.

Events Following World War II

During the 1940s and 1950s (1945–59)

The events during the fifteen years that followed V-J Day brought more areas of change more rapidly than did any other period in the history of nursing. Health care systems in the United States were viewed differently after the war. The public became more aware of what constitutes good health care, the population increased, and the economy changed and grew. There was a trend toward urbanization, an explosion of scientific knowledge, an acceleration of medical discoveries, new methods of therapy, new inventions, and finally, the recognition that it is just as important to keep people well as it is to treat illness. After World War II an effort was made to move more deliberately and more creatively; the impact of this movement continues to be felt with increasing intensity.

As knowledge increased and the economy changed, there were new developments in education. For instance, the GI Bill of Rights had a major impact; numerous veterans could now prepare for careers for which they, at one time, had never dreamed they could qualify. All schools, including nursing schools, were flooded with applicants for degrees. Education was changing the practice of nursing.

One theme heard frequently during the postwar era was, "The nurse must give total patient care." Nurses were to be all things to their clients. Although other health team members were present, nurses were either reluctant to give up the idea of *total patient care,* or perhaps did not know how to relinquish the aspects of care that were not nursing. The scene began to change and the nurse learned that teamwork was the name of the new game. It was not easy for her to relinquish the idea that she had to be all things to all clients. Gradually emphasis shifted, and although the nurse continued to be aware of the totality of the individual client, her role was altered to include working cooperatively with other members of the health team who were also concerned with the client's care and welfare. Referral of clients to members of other disciplines became the nurse's responsibility. She continued the concept of total patient care; however, implementation of the concept was now the responsibility of the entire health team, including the nurse. Communication also became the responsibility of all health team members.

The war precipitated changes during the early 1940s, and the later years of this decade witnessed a concerned nursing profession. Health care personnel were struggling with the increased number of people who had been introduced into the health care system. Roles were defined to prevent duplication, yet each group tried to retain the essence of its own role as its members perceived it. The changes in nursing created turmoil that culminated, finally, in asking a nonnurse to provide an unbiased assessment of the status of the profession and to suggest ways in which it could move constructively. The report presented by Esther Lucile Brown in 1948 was a major turning point in the lives of nurses and in nursing.[3]

The groundwork provided by the recommendations of this report was the basis for many of the changes in nursing during the next thirty years.

As did Florence Nightingale, Esther Brown expressed her concern for adequate remuneration of nurses for quality service. Significantly, the discussion of remuneration seldom stood alone; it was usually coupled with mention of the responsibility for providing quality service. This concern is as true today as it was in the days of Florence Nightingale, and it is one of the major justifications for employing the nursing process. Through organized and deliberate nursing action, provision of quality care is more certain, and the means for evaluating the quality of care are provided.

During the 1950s, after the Brown report was published, much attention was focused on the appropriate use of the term *professional.* For many years professionalism had been discussed and there were debates about whether or not nursing met the criteria for a profession. Several authors suggested criteria for a profession; those stated by Flexner [4] were quoted frequently. More recently, several sociologists identified the variables that operate in defining professionalism and establishing criteria basic to professions. Schein presented a composite of these efforts and delineated ten criteria of professions, all of which are appropriate to the profession of nursing.[5]

During the latter part of the 1950s, attempts were made to define nursing functions in relation to professional activities. When nursing actions were discussed, a number of crucial questions were asked, such as: To what extent do the actions of the nurse affect people? How significant are her decisions and judgments to the present and the future welfare of the service consumer? How complex are these actions in terms of the nurse's education and experience? Is there ample and appropriate knowledge available to and used by the nurse as a basis for her acts? Is there some check on the effectiveness of her actions? Does her performance improve with experience, and does she modify her plans according to available knowledge and experience? Is the consumer able to judge the effectiveness of a nursing action? He can judge it in terms of his own needs, but is this the only measure available to him? How does a specific act compare with similar actions of other nurses? [6]

Inherent within these criteria and questions is the pertinent observation that a code of ethics is both important and essential. The most recent revision of the Code of Ethics for nurses stresses self-determination of clients, the nurse's role as patient advocate, and the need for quality assurance and peer review.[7] Such a code is important because it meets one criterion for a profession. More important, however, is the use of a code in practice and the perception of the statements within the code as legitimate guidelines to direct the nurse–client relationship.

Nurses continue to be concerned that nursing should meet the criteria for a profession; however, nursing actions and the client who is the recipient of nursing are receiving increased emphasis, rather than the nurse who does, or who is, the agent of nursing. Nurses, themselves, generally view nursing as a profession; as a group of professionals, their major concern is to provide quality care for clients, and energies are devoted to determining the best means to provide the best care.

During the 1960s and 1970s (1960–78)

One of the major events of the 1960s was the publication of the *American Nurses' Association's First Position on Education for Nursing*. The position paper, which initiated many discussions and debates, is indicative of a definite trend in nursing. Essentially, the position of the American Nurses' Association is that the education of persons who practice nursing should take place in institutions of higher education; the professional nurse should be prepared in baccalaureate programs of nursing, the technical nurse in associate degree programs, and the assistant in the health services in preservice programs in vocational education institutions rather than in on-the-job training programs.[8]

The position paper was not precipitous. It resulted from a study that covered more than a ten-year period, which was conducted by the ANA Committee on Current and Long-Term Goals and the ANA Committee on Education. The turmoil among nurses who reacted to the position paper has been long-lived. Some short-sighted nurses fail to see the importance of educational preparation; others continue to approve the pursuit of education over a prolonged time. The reality of nursing is, however, that ". . . whether it suits us personally or not, education for nursing must be at least as encompassing and as rigorous as that for other professions."[9]

Another significant event was the appointment, in 1961, by the surgeon general of the United States Public Health Service, of the Consultant Group on Nursing that was to provide advice about nursing needs and problems in the United States. The group operated on the basis that nursing is an essential element in health care, and that public understanding and support will be necessary to solve problems in nursing. Although the group was concerned with an increasing demand for nurses, the need for quality in nursing education, nursing service, and nursing research was constantly emphasized. The group identified needs and set goals for nursing during the 1970s.[10] The recommendations of this study led to the appointment of the National Commission for the Study of Nursing and Nursing Education. The appointed commissioners met for the first time in 1967. A comprehensive and in-depth study resulted from the efforts of the members of this commission; they pursued three areas: nursing roles and functions, nursing education, and professional growth and development. Specific recommendations related to increased research, altered educational patterns, and enhanced support for nursing are contained in the report.[11] The efforts of the consultant group and the commissioners further emphasize the importance of pursuing nursing in a systematic way, so that deliberate goal-directed activity is the focus of nursing and evaluation of goal achievement is possible.

Many factors contributed to the turmoil and unrest felt by society during the 1960s and 1970s. The riots on college campuses in the sixties, the emphasis on human rights in the seventies, and other aspects of this period require extensive study and analysis to be completely understood. Many of the changes in education, and especially the practice of nursing, were outgrowths of the societal events of the day.

One significant event in nursing was the trend toward "independent practice," which began as a concept during the 1960s and developed into action in the 1970s.[12,13] Although the role of nursing practitioner is growing during the 1970s, not all who function as practitioners perform nursing in like manner. Some function independently as generalists; others set up group practice, utilizing the special talents of several nurses; still others function within the established health system and/or with a physician or group of physicians. Some practitioners pursue special programs to develop skills and expertise they need to fill a role they have identified. Other practitioners rely on already acquired knowledge and skills. An important positive result of this development in nursing is the emergence of nurses who now perceive their role as nurse in a self-supporting way. This is a role that is not dependent on any other discipline or profession for viability, but is sufficient unto itself in providing nursing for clients in the form of professional actions based on sound judgments.

In addition, the number of nurses who are pursuing preparation beyond the basic program in nursing and who are developing skills in research and systematic study is increasing. By means of such expertise, sophisticated data will be added to the nursing knowledge that is already available; nurses and clients will continually benefit from such professional advances.

The emphasis on maintenance of wellness in addition to care of persons who are ill allows nurses entry into many settings to provide health care and presents the opportunities for a variety of role performances. The potential areas for quality nursing are truly increasing with better prepared nurses who have an expanded vision of their health care opportunities.

Licensure of the professional and practical nurse continues to be of concern, and its relation to continuing education is most complex. Several jurisdictions are experimenting with different plans that will provide continuing education units for each nurse when and if such credentialing becomes mandatory. In reference to the licensure question, the most recent event that created much debate and dialogue is the effort by the New York State Nurses' Association to require by 1985 a baccalaureate degree for licensure as a professional nurse and an associate degree for licensure as a practical nurse.[14] The topic was deliberated at the ANA Biennial Convention in June 1976, and it was suggested that a national conference be called in which issues would be discussed and positions would be identified.[15] At the end of 1976 it was announced that the American Nurses' Association had launched a major study of credentialing in nursing; a study to be completed in a 22-month period so that outcomes could be presented at the 1978 ANA Convention. The study will assess current credentialing mechanisms including certification, licensure, and accreditation of basic, graduate, continuing education, and organized nursing service programs.[16]

Although the vista of nursing is expanding, it is obvious that nurses continue to disagree about some of the basics, for example, the assigning of appropriate labels to use to describe the actions performed in the new settings. Are the nurses to be known as nurse practitioners? Nursing practitioners?[17] Independent practitioners? Generalists? Specialists? Primary nurses? Clinicians? Language and labels are important and clarification of the terms used by nurses will continue to be a challenge in the future,[18] but this concern for labels should not impede the forward thrust of nursing practice.

The 1960s and 1970s are decades of excitement and change. A selected few of the significant events of these decades have been mentioned and briefly summarized. The challenge of coping with the complex climate in which nurses function today is both staggering and stimulating. Within the numerous events, however, one movement has grown and flourished: the Nursing Process. Continued development is expected; nursing is coming of age.

Definitions of Nursing

The definition of nursing developed by each nurse may vary according to the language used, the setting one has in mind, and the personal orientation of the nurse based on her education and experience.

One can read any definition of nursing and assume or interpret the author's thoughts and intent. For example, the word *patient* can suggest that the author thinks of a person who is sick or not well and for whom she is responsible. This need not, but frequently does, exclude the preventive aspect of nursing.

The settings for nursing suggest that adaptability is necessary to cope with present situations. Journeys into space make extraterrestrial nursing a possibility; it can no longer be regarded as fictional. Until space stations are constructed and put into operation, however, nursing needs on the planet earth are many and varied. The client who is the potential and actual recipient of nursing exists in a number of environs. Preventive and therapeutic nursing are needed in any setting; the intensity of the need varies with the degree or extent to which the service is needed, the time at which the client enters the health care system, and the place or setting in which he finds himself when the need for service arises.

Another variable in defining nursing is the breadth and depth of vision held by the nurse regarding the service she is able to provide. If her vision is myopic, she will provide a much different quality of service than the broad-visioned operator or agent. As one grows in maturity, in life, and in work experience, one sees himself or herself and others more clearly, with more potential than when younger and less experienced. Each age has its merits, and a delicious blend of vigorous youth and healthy ripening or flowering maturity is a desirable mixture. Each learns from the other and benefits from open-minded exchanges to the ultimate benefit of the recipient of nursing, the client.

Despite variations in definitions of nursing, individuals and groups of nurses should continue to strive to assemble words that represent their ideas and reflect the service of nursing as they see it. This would seem to be more important than continuing to look for one definition of nursing that will be universally accepted. Synonyms, in any language, allow for a number of words, any one, or any combination of which, can be used to describe the service nurses provide. A variety of resources can be used, including each concerned nurse, to describe nursing; the definition of nursing is then expressed as a foundation for functioning. The nurse is then ready to move to the essential actions of nursing, for which the definition is the springboard or beginning.

Although the literature contains materials about the question, What is nursing?, perhaps the answer is so obvious that a precise definition is unnecessary or the many operant variables make a precise definition impossible. Most nursing texts contain at least one sizeable section in which nursing is defined as it is perceived by the author(s). Nurses appear ready to accept, respect, and expect nurse-authors as well as nurse-practitioners to present their individual definitions and concepts about nursing.

When the structure of society was less complex than it is today, the intuitive functioning of the nurse was usually adequate to provide care. A well-intentioned, well-meaning person with an innate ability to care for the sick was an excellent person to help those who were ill. Even in that uncomplicated day, however, each person had a different mental image of the term *nursing*. Today, a number of variables determine the complexion of this image, ranging from the actions of a mother surrogate to those of a top-level administrator. The discussion of *what is nursing* can be approached from any one of a number of avenues. Nursing can be defined or discussed according to the actions used in performing the service; the roles of the persons who do the nursing; the functions of the nurse; the consumer's image of nursing; the image of nursing held by nursing peers; the philosophy of nursing as perceived by practitioners; the settings where nursing is performed; the value placed on the individual who needs nursing; and respect for the client viewed from the employer-employee standpoint. One can begin to discuss or to define nursing from such points. These potential areas are mentioned to emphasize the complex nature of nursing.

A number of nurses have defined nursing; some have defined a concept of nursing, others have stated beliefs about nursing, still others have defined a philosophy of nursing, and several have discussed theory and nursing. Important data referring to these subjects can be found in nursing publications, all of which are attempts to state the essence of nursing.

Some nurses have contributed to the efforts to define nursing, each developing and making a statement as to what nursing is based on her own philosophy, education, and experience. Throughout these efforts to define the unique function of nursing, various authors have expressed, in different words, what they see as the function and role of nursing. It is apparent that there is something different about nursing than the service provided by other disciplines. Some suggest that the uniqueness of nursing may be the ability to use data from other disciplines. Although many nurses have developed definitions of nursing independently, the various presentations convey similar ideas but use different words and various frames of reference. Individual values are apparent in each definition; one can determine the extent to which a client is viewed as a person and the extent to which he is respected as an individual with human needs and human rights. These are guides used by the nurse to define and report what it is she finds important in nursing.

To illustrate the development of ideas about nursing, several selected discussions about definitions of nursing are presented.

One of the earliest definitions of nursing was presented in 1943 by Sister Olivia Gowan, a far-sighted pioneer in nursing education. Sister viewed nursing, in its broadest sense, as being both an art and a science involving the total patient; as promoting spiritual, mental, and physical health; stressing health education and health preservation; ministering to the sick; caring for the patient's environment; and as giving health service to the family, the community, and the individual.[19] This definition appeared in print long before it was fashionable to define nursing, and the comprehensive definition of nursing given by Sister Olivia was, for many years, most accepted and often quoted. Long recognized as an outstanding leader in nursing, Sister died in April, 1977.

Another respected leader in nursing, Francis Reiter Kreuter, died in January, 1977. An article in *Nursing Outlook* in 1957, in which Kreuter [20] discussed good nursing care, is frequently referred to by nurses. Certain themes and concepts are evident as one reads her material, especially her vision of the nurse as the mother surrogate. Not all nurses agree with this interpretation of their role, but if one analyzes Erikson's identification of the developmental phases of childhood and the role of the parent in each phase, the term *mother surrogate* becomes more acceptable. For example, a basic tenet in teaching a child is to gain his or her trust; so too, trust in the nurse is the basis for the client care she provides. A child learns independence gradually; the mother teaches him and helps him to become independent as he grows and develops. Developing initiative is fostered and encouraged by the mother so that the child can progress to the limit of his abilities.[21] These findings can be applied to the roles of nurse and client, in which Kreuter saw the nurse as protecting the patient, teaching him, performing for him those acts of self-care he cannot do himself, and providing comfort and encouragement. Although she called these "ministrations," they can also be viewed as nursing actions–ministering to basic needs, administering, observing, teaching, supervising, or guiding, planning with, and communicating with the patient. Kreuter also discussed direct care, in which the nurse gives direct physical care, and indirect care, in which she engages in activities that do not bring her into immediate contact with the client. Some nurses agree with these concepts in their entirety; some agree with them partially; nevertheless, Kreuter made major contributions to the development of concepts of nursing through numerous and thought-provoking materials.

Dorothy Johnson's presentations have also precipitated thought and discussion among nurses. Central to her thesis is the idea that all health workers have something unique to offer the client, but how to determine that which is uniquely nursing is the question that concerns nurses. To cope with the client's problems, each person sees certain nursing problems that require assessment, decision, and action.[22] Dr. Johnson suggests that nursing is a direct service to persons under stress relative to their basic human needs.[23] Nursing effort and actions are focused on relieving tension and establishing interpersonal equilibrium. This equilibrium is a dynamic and transitional state in which stability is a delicately balanced component. Once stability is achieved, constant adjustment and effort are necessary to maintain it. The activities in which nurses are engaged for the benefit of the client should contribute to the goal of equilibrium.[23]

In 1963, Ernestine Wiedenbach contributed additional ideas to the nursing literature. She identified the purpose of nursing as meeting the requirements of persons experiencing some need for help. Three major units of nursing practice were identified: (a) recognizing a person's need for help, (b) giving or ministering that help, and (c) validating that the help given was the help needed. The heart of nursing was seen as the act of helping others; due concern was expressed for the nurse's feelings and thoughts as well as for those of the client experiencing the problem. Essentially, emphasis was placed on the interpersonal aspect of actions that are nursing, and on identifying the behavioral stimulus for the person in need so as to designate the actions to take. The purpose of nursing was identified as "facilitating the efforts of the individual to overcome obstacles which interfere with his ability to respond capably to demands made of him by his condition, environment, situation, and time." [24]

Although she identified her ideas and concepts much earlier than 1966, Virginia Henderson's book, *The Nature of Nursing,* published that year, contributed data to the increasing growth of information about nursing. Certain ideas and thoughts were distinctive about Miss Henderson's writings. She urged each nurse to define, for herself, what she sees nursing to be and to develop her own concept, rather than merely imitate others or act under the pressure of authority. The nurse was viewed as an independent practitioner, helping the client to perform those activities he could not perform unaided at a given time. Miss Henderson was one of the few persons to include in her definition the idea that efforts to return the client to a state of wellness are not always successful. She recognized that unless a nurse is realistic about the probable or possible negative outcome of a client's illness, she will be prone to disappointment and frustration. However, if the nurse includes in her role the responsibility to help the client achieve a peaceful death, both client and nurse will recognize their roles more precisely and be able to set realistic goals for themselves. Miss Henderson states, "The unique function of the nurse is to assist the individual, sick or well, in the performance of these activities contributing to health or its recovery (or to peaceful death) that he would perform unaided if he had the necessary strength, will, or knowledge." [25] The focus of nursing actions, according to Henderson, is to provide physical care for clients. The definition of this care can be interpreted broadly to include intellectual, interpersonal, and technical activities. Miss Henderson's discussions of nursing and her illustrations of nursing functions suggest that she views nursing in this broad context.

These few examples of published concepts about nursing serve to emphasize Catherine Norris' contention that a major delusion in nursing is that nurses agree about what nursing is.[26] She pointedly identifies the multiple dimensions of the dilemma that nurses face, suggesting that "the support of a theoretical frame of reference" is needed in order to better develop the "processes of history taking and nursing assessment, diagnosis, and intervention which are still in primitive stages of development." [27]

A conscious awareness of one's personal philosophy and due consideration for human values, ethics, and beliefs are essential if one wishes to develop his or her own definition of nursing and refute some of the delusions posed by Norris. Therefore, the authors present the following definition on which the content of this text is based: *Nursing is an encounter with a client and his family in which the nurse observes, supports, communicates, ministers, and teaches; she contributes to the maintenance of optimum health, and provides care during illness until the client is able to assume responsibility for the fulfillment of his own basic human needs; when necessary, she provides compassionate assistance with dying.*

A review of nursing literature reveals that efforts have been made during the past 15 years to state a definition of nursing that can be accepted as universally as that given by Sister Olivia Gowan. Gradually, however, concern over a definition of nursing is being diluted by attempts to develop theoretical frameworks and theories that underlie nursing, and to define concepts that make nursing what it is, that is, to clarify the art and science of nursing in the light of increasing knowledge in related biologic and behavioral fields.

Knowledge continues to grow at a faster pace than it did during the immediate postwar years. Technology and computers, progress in education, and the space age have had an overwhelming impact on the forward momentum of advances and changes in today's society. The layman began to be heard more clearly after the world survived the second world war. The public has become more knowledgeable, is learning more and more about its health, its illnesses, and its rights; the vocal client is not only presenting new challenges to the health professions, but is also creating a need for new approaches to health care, emphasizing the need for preventive medicine as well as therapeutic care during sickness.

History records significant events in the development of nursing, and these can be grouped according to those that occurred before, during, and after World War II. Nursing moved from a humanitarian caring for the sick, through a period of complacency, and survived the acceleration of all facets of life as well as changes in the health scene precipitated by and following World War II. The Brown Report in 1948, the ANA Position Paper in 1965, the Report of the Surgeon General's Consultant Group, and the report of the National Commission to Study Nursing and Nursing Education in 1970 are major events that have stimulated changes in nursing. Having survived efforts to prove that nursing is a profession and verbal barrages in attempts to define nursing and what is unique about it, the profession is now seriously involved in defining the theoretical and conceptual frameworks for nursing.

Philosophy, Theory, Concept, Process

Philosophy, theory, concept, and process are components of nursing on and around which nursing is built. A sound philosophy with clearly expressed values and beliefs provides a foundation for nursing. Identification of theories and the pursuit of those having significance for nursing are continuing activities as scientific foundations are established. Theories from various disciplines are utilized and adopted as the development of a nursing science is pursued and as nurses rely on already established data as a base for their actions. Newly identified concepts add to the knowledge and use of theories, and the process of nursing relies on all of these firm bases to assure sound practice. Intellectual, interpersonal, and technical skills are used in the application of the nursing process by the nurse as she performs actions for the client based on identified theories and concepts.

The identification and clarification of these terms will continue to be discussed and deliberated by professional nurses. To add to the challenge, the nurse has the option of choosing either the inductive or the deductive means of exploration. Some nurses prefer the inductive method, that is, identification of nurse actions in the client care arena and definition of concepts and theories employed in nursing that are derived from those actions. Other nurses find the deductive method more effective, i.e., first, the definition of theories, then a description of the concepts that constitute those theories, and finally the citation, in the client action arena, of those parts of the process performed within appropriate concepts and theories. Either approach can be legitimately pursued; hopefully, both approaches will be followed by different nurses, in different settings, and on a continuous basis, to assist in the validation of acquired data.

To synonymously use a statement of one's philosophy, to label the same statement as both a theory and a concept, and to indiscriminately use the nursing process label to cover all actions for the client suggests that these terms are used ambiguously in nursing. A brief presentation of some means to differentiate each term will assist the reader in understanding the authors' views of these terms. More reading, studying, and discussion with peers and others will be necessary to fully appreciate the significance of these terms that are so crucial to nursing.

Philosophy

In a strict sense, philosophy is a science unto itself, a "science of beings in terms of their ultimate causes." [28] The value of the science of philosophy is to assist persons to direct their activities by reflecting on the essence of who they are and what they are. In this sense, nurses utilize a philosophic base to express their orientation about man and the universe in which persons who are clients may need the assistance of others, who may be nurses.

Philosophers Dickoff and James have engaged in stimulating dialogues with nurses about nursing over a period of time and have differentiated between the nurse's and the philosopher's approach: "What nurses tend to call 'philosophy of nursing' we as philosophers would tend to call . . . a 'religion of nursing'."[29] To Dickoff and James, philosophy is "an approach, not a set of beliefs."[29] Whether labeled as a "philosophy of nursing" or a "set of beliefs," each nurse possesses a set of inherent values. She has certain beliefs about man, his purpose in life, and his destiny. These beliefs direct the manner by which persons relate to each other, the way they work with each other, and the way they care for those who need or can benefit from their nursing actions. An awareness and understanding of one's own philosophy and values and a deliberate expression of one's beliefs about man are fundamental to the performance of quality nursing.

Theory

A theory is a systematically related set of statements that describes, explains, and predicts parts of the empirical, or real, world. This set of statements may include some law-like generalizations that can be tested in reality.[30] Theories are also known as bodies of generalizations developed in association with practice, and these data form the intellectual aspect of a discipline.[31] Theory can be called an hypothesis, involving some interesting ideas or opinions.[32] Central to a variety of definitions of theory, and significant to the relationship of theory to nursing are these elements: theories are abstractions, they are generalizations, and they are related to practice.

Perhaps one of the unique features of nursing is the use of knowledge from various disciplines to perform the actions of client care. Theories from various biopsychosocial sciences have potential use in nursing, several of which can be identified; for example, from sociology, one can identify facets of a sociologic framework for client care. Theories from the biologic sciences may be more pertinent for the client with a physiologic health deficit. Basing client care on known theories from the biopsychosocial sciences is a legitimate manner of establishing a framework for client care.

Theories, then, are broad, encompass a number of ideas, and are influential in directing the nursing care of clients. They are abstract and intangible, but must have some basis in practice to be legitimately recognized as nursing theories. A theory for the sake of theory alone provides an exercise for the pure scientist. The nurse is concerned about the practical science of nursing. Therefore, theory in nursing will be selected and used with some relationship to practice.

The need for sound theories to guide the practice of nursing has been expressed many times. Basic scientific theories can be identified, tested, and evaluated while the nurse deliberately cares for clients. From the planned actions of the practitioner, theories that guide actions can be retested and reexplored to assess their value and the extent to which they help to improve the practice of nursing. "Hunches" can be defined and ideas used to pursue further theories and actions, thereby establishing a continual cycle of activity—selecting a theory, using a theory to prescribe and plan nursing, testing the effectiveness of the action in terms of benefit to the client, revising, redefining, perhaps determining a new or selecting a different theory to use, and testing and reevaluating for future actions. The deliberate use of theories, therefore, assists in the sound planning and implementation of nursing actions, and results in quality nursing practice. Nurses have relied on the related disciplines to define theories on which nursing actions and roles can be based. Persons in the behavioral and physical science disciplines have been generous in providing assistance to the nursing profession. Results of an investigation, conducted under a research grant from the National Institute of Mental Health, prompted sociologists Johnson and Martin to propose one type of theoretical base. They did not seek to solve all problems of nursing, but proposed a means by which nurses could view and analyze what they were doing. First, they hypothesized that any social system has certain functional responsibilities, which they defined as: (a) making progress toward the defined goal or purpose for which the group exists; and (b) maintaining harmonious relationships among group members so that internal equilibrium can be maintained and the group will be cohesive and integrated. Actions to direct the group toward achieving its goals are called *instrumental actions;* actions for the purpose of maintaining equilibrium of group members are called *expressive actions.*[33] The investigation itself focused primarily on the functioning of group members and secondly on the recipients of group action. The theoretical base derived from this study can be applied to nursing in the following way: as members of the health team direct their efforts toward treating the client who is ill, their functions and actions are said to be instrumental. To achieve the desired goal of helping the client to recover, communication among health team members, as well as collaboration and sharing of plans, ideas, and efforts is necessary. The more effective the group is in maintaining a spirit of cooperation among its members, the more likely it is to achieve its goal of providing the client with the best care; these latter functions are termed expressive actions. Deliberate awareness of these differences in roles will assist in a more orderly and systematic analysis of nursing actions.

Just as there has been a gradual but sure movement in nursing away from instinctive performance of actions, so has there been an effort to identify the intellectual aspect of nursing that directs the actions of the nurse. Efforts are also being made to close the gap existing between the art and the science of nursing, or the practice and theory of nursing. The goal of the science of nursing is defined as understanding, whereas that of the art of nursing is defined as skill, according to McKay.[34] The art and the science of nursing are integral parts of the nursing process. Science suggests knowledge, or intellectualization; art suggests action. "In the nursing process, both intelligence and technique are needed and, in addition, values must be upheld."[34]

Concept

Concepts are general notions,[32] thoughts, ideas[31]; they are descriptive terms.[30] Like theories, concepts are intangible. A number of concepts may comprise a theory. For example, conceptual terms may be used to describe tangible objects, such as green, soft material. One cannot touch greenness or softness, but one can describe what each looks or feels like. Both characteristics apply to one piece of material, however. Concepts are essential elements that make up the theory; thus they are less broad than theory but more broad than process.

In one study, Horgan searched the nursing literature to determine what concepts existed.[35] Thirty concepts were found in two professional nursing periodicals from 1950 to 1965. Twelve concepts appeared between 1950 and 1960. Eighteen concepts appeared between 1960 and 1965. One of Horgan's assumptions is that concepts about nursing and the nursing process share components and elements in common. She defined a concept of nursing as "an expression in words by the author of the ideas, which summarize the elements and components of what she thinks about nursing and the nursing process, or some aspect of this process." She concluded with the observation that nursing concepts were person- and action-centered; the persons were named by position—nurse and patient. Action was described as meeting patients' needs or as the nurse's initiating a system or process to assess, fulfill, and validate the action necessary to meet patients' needs. Many of the concepts were not general; they were limited to specific stages or aspects of nursing or to a specific condition of the patient. The concepts did not emphasize the general health needs of people or nursing as a health service in society. The ultimate goals of nursing seemed to be in meeting the needs of patients. Concepts seemed to center on the technology of assessing and validating needs, not on their fulfillment.

Since 1965, when Horgan's study was completed, there has been a marked increase in publications by nurses about concepts, nursing concepts, and conceptual frameworks.[36-45] Some differences of opinion still exist about theories and concepts. Not all agree about what each term really means, about how one differs from another, how each is used in nursing, and why the use of the theories and concepts will improve the quality of client care. It is encouraging, however, to witness the growth in the number of explorations and deliberations in this area and also to note the increasing quality of the publications by persons who are exploring and using theories and concepts in nursing.

Process

Process is an act of moving forward, or progressing from one point to another on the way to completion of a goal; it is the continuous movement through a succession of developmental stages; it is the method by which something is produced, something is accomplished, or a specific result is attained; it is an act that continues, or progresses.[31] Process is also a change, using feedback, as one proceeds toward an objective.[46] The central ideas in these definitions suggest that when one is concerned with process, there is movement in a forward direction, and the continued movement is based on data collected from the person who should benefit from the action being done.

The perception of a process as an action suggests a power behind the action or a mover of the action, hence control and/or systematic movement. Conscious and deliberate effort must be exerted to arrive at a defined goal. The absence of a planned or deliberate movement results in a mechanical effort, perhaps chaotic in nature, and certainly not orderly or systematic. Absence of a goal toward which a process is directed has the potential of rendering that process useless; it has no meaning if there is no purpose or potential for application. The basic idea of a process is that it is a unit; it can be described as consisting of phases, but each phase is dependent on the others—none stands alone. The elements can be distinguished for analysis and scrutiny, but for useful and practical purposes, a total understanding of process is necessary.

The *nursing process is an orderly, systematic manner of determining the client's problems, making plans to solve them, initiating the plan or assigning others to implement it, and evaluating the extent to which the plan was effective in resolving the problems identified.*

Leadership, Research, Nursing Processes

The leadership process, the research process, and the nursing process form an important triad in nursing. Although there are similarities among the three processes, each has its own specific purpose and distinct goals. Nurses use the three processes in caring for clients and their families.

The leadership process involves decision making, relating, influencing, and facilitating, with the ultimate goal of directing a group to achieve a defined goal.[47]

The research process involves collecting and analyzing data and reaching conclusions, with the ultimate goal of discovering new knowledge about a situation.[48]

The nursing process involves assessing, planning, implementing, and evaluating client situations, with the ultimate goal of preventing or resolving problematic situations.

Required Nursing Skills

The nurse uses many skills in the pursuit of nursing. The skills necessary for the conduct of the nursing process can be categorized into three groups, namely, intellectual, interpersonal, and technical skills.

Intellectual skills are those that form the knowledge component of nursing. Acquired data from educational and life experiences give each nurse a basis for making decisions, arriving at judgments, and setting priorities. Drawing conclusions based on intellectual data enables the nurse to move deliberately and with certainty rather than instinctively and haphazardly. The laws and principles employed in the pursuit of nursing form a sound basis against which actions can be examined, validated, and repeated as necessary. Despite the rapid increase in knowledge available in the twentieth century, and the establishment of a reasonable framework for performing nursing, nurses can make increasingly constructive use of data available to them and can continually add to the intellectual component of nursing.

The *interpersonal skills* of the nurse are those that deal with relating to the client as a person, to his family and/or significant others, to the community from which he comes, the community in which his care is being given, to the other health disciplines associated with his care, and to the nursing personnel responsible for his nursing care. The interpersonal skills necessary for nursing have multiple dimensions.

To use the nursing process in the desired manner, each nurse must develop certain behaviors to make her efforts more effective so that the client will receive better care. Her innate abilities and acquired knowledge will be fundamental to any nursing performance. The interpersonal techniques one learns throughout life enable the nurse to know herself and to deal with others. Dealing effectively with others presents a continuing challenge that usually motivates and stimulates the nurse to think in terms of coping with each individual. To achieve qualitative results, nursing behavior should include problem-solving orientation, and problem-solving techniques should be developed deliberately.[49]

Certain behaviors will prove to be more successful than others in helping the nurse to use her abilities and knowledge. Creativity, adaptability, commitment, trust, and leadership are characteristics or behaviors conducive to better performance of nursing actions that comprise the nursing process.

In judging which actions are necessary to assist the client with his problems, the nurse uses her skills of perception, observation, and communication.

Perception suggests insight into various facets of a situation. The nurse develops insight into what she sees as a client's problem, into what she hears the client say he needs, and into how these data relate to each other. The nurse reflects on similar situations she has encountered in the past, on the significance and meaning of various cues she perceives, and on the variety of human factors she is able to identify in the situation. Foresight is also necessary. As the nurse observes the client's immediate status, she is thinking of his future. For example, an instrument maker who enters the emergency room with a relatively serious injury to his thumb will have immediate needs; with her immediate actions, the nurse simultaneously thinks of the questions that will arise: Will job adjustment be necessary? How soon will prognosis be known? What can he be told if he asks about prognosis?

The art of communication includes talking as well as listening. Communication with the client begins with the first face-to-face contact between him and the nurse. A deliberately worded greeting and careful listening to the client's reply will set the stage for a good encounter.

Adaptability suggests that the nurse is able to adapt to whatever situation she encounters; she is able to adjust to varying demands of the same or several situations; she is able to employ acceptable and appropriate means to provide care for various clients with different backgrounds and individual idiosyncrasies. This suggests that she has a plan rather than entering the situation unprepared. She validates her perceptions with the client and makes plans with him, adjusting and changing them when necessary. Adaptability suggests flexibility, with enough structure to promote the process of nursing.

The successful nurse is the committed nurse. She is the person who sees the client as an individual and respects his humanity, his rights, his beliefs, and his interest in himself. Concern for herself is a part of the committed nurse's interest; however, this self-concern is intended to promote more careful self-assessment so that she can become more aware of her own abilities and limitations. This in turn will make her more capable of dealing with client concerns and needs. A good portion of selflessness is inherent in the committed nurse's actions.

Mutual trust is essential in the care of any client. Only when the client feels that the nurse trusts him will he be able to share needed information with her. Any sense of distrust will destroy this relationship, once it has been established, or any potential relationship. Just as the client must be able to trust the nurse, so the nurse must be able to trust the client. Honesty in dealing with each other will encourage this mutual trust relationship and, once established, it will be a solid foundation on which to build future and further encounters.

Leadership is a desirable trait in pursuit of the nursing process. Personal abilities and healthy initiative foster the development of a model of desirable behavior, which is needed to pursue the nursing process. With capable leadership qualities, the nurse initiates changes, uses creativity, and performs as a role model to promote a sense of trust and a feeling of commitment, and utilizes adaptability in an effective way.

Technical Skills in the past have often been the only skills associated with the process of nursing. The nurse was perceived as a "doer"; she performed actions and was the initiator as well as the one who continued the activities of client care; she was historically the only one who did what was necessary for nursing care.

The technical aspect of nursing continues to be an essential component in nursing. However, it is not the total nursing process, nor is nursing the only discipline responsible for "doing" for the client. Depending on the needs of the client and the setting where care is being provided, the utilization of technical skills by the nurse will vary. For example, the client in an intensive care unit of a hospital requires sophisticated technical nursing skills; a client who is dying at home requires astute and compassionate technical nursing skills.

Throughout the application of the nursing process, a reasonable use of each skill and due attention to the three skills, intellectual, interpersonal, and technical, will insure more qualitative utilization of the nursing process and more satisfactory completion of quality client care.

History of the Nursing Process

From its embryonic stage in the 1950s, the nursing process has now become a readily recognized and well-used activity. A review of a few of the recent developments in nursing reveals the rate at which the nursing process reached its present stage of development.

In 1955, Lydia Hall spoke to a group of nurses in New Jersey about the quality of nursing care. Having once heard Mrs. Hall speak to a group, few could forget her unique platform style. The content of her presentation to the New Jersey group was unforgettable, too. She discussed her ideas about nursing, then stated the assumption basic to her total presentation: "Nursing is a process." She defined the use of four prepositions that indicate a relationship to, and that can be used to describe the range in quality of, the nursing process from not so good to very good. The four prepositions are: Nursing *at* the patient, *to* the patient, *for* the patient, and *with* the patient.[50]

Orlando's text was published at the beginning of the 1960s. It has been referred to frequently for its presentation of the nursing process as well as for its differentiation of nursing activities. The central focus of Orlando's text, *The Dynamic Nurse-Patient Relationship*, is the interpersonal relationship.[51] A proponent of deliberative actions, Orlando distinguished them from automatic activities that can become part of the nurse's functioning. She was as concerned for the client and his needs as were others who wrote about nursing. Orlando was one of the earliest authors to use the term *the nursing process.* Although others used the words, none had discussed the process in the same detail as did Orlando, nor had nurses been attracted to the label until the early years of the 1960s. Despite this pioneering effort, the term was not adopted immediately. Orlando identified a nursing situation as comprising three elements: (a) behavior of the patient, (b) reaction of the nurse, and (c) nursing actions designed for the patient's benefit. The interaction of these elements with each other is the nursing process.[51] Although attention was directed to the interpersonal aspect of care, appropriate attention to the physical and social aspects of care is included in the discussion of the process. As did others who defined nursing and identified concepts of nursing, due attention was given to environmental influences as well as to variables inherent in different settings in which nurses care for clients.

While Lydia Hall saw nursing as a process and Orlando defined phases of the process in terms of interpersonal relationships, other nurses were exploring ways of analyzing their philosophy and values.

In 1966, Lois Knowles presented a description of a model of the activities in which the nurse is engaged.[52] She suggested that the nurse's success as a practitioner depends on her mastery of the five D's: (a) Discover–she acquires knowledge or information about something that she did not know previously; such information should contribute to better client care. (b) Delve–she derives information from as many sources as possible to provide data about the client, which will assist her in providing for his care. (c) Decide –she plans the approach to use in the client's care. All facets of the problems are considered and the best course of action is designed. (d) Do–she administers, performs, and activates the plan that has been developed. (e) Discriminate–she distinguishes priorities and reactions by discerning differences in problems and the needs experienced by the client. Although not identical to phases of the nursing process as identified herein, these five D's suggest another way of approaching client care.[52]

In 1967, a committee involved with curriculum development in the western states defined the nursing process as ". . . that which goes on between a patient and nurse in a given setting; it incorporates the behaviors of patient and nurse and the resulting interaction. The steps in the process are: perception, communication, interpretation, intervention, and evaluation." [53] Also, in 1967, a faculty group at the school of nursing at The Catholic University of America identified the phases of the nursing process as: assessing, planning, implementing, and evaluating.[54]

Few studies in nursing have been conducted in the same manner as the extensive research project undertaken by an interdisciplinary group at the University of Colorado; the results were reported in a series of articles published in *Nursing Research* over a period of time.[55-61] The purpose of the study was to investigate the clinical inference process as it referred to nursing. The responsibility of inferring the patient's needs was viewed as making judgments about the patient based on available data. Essentially, this can be interpreted as diagnosing the client's problems. When the client has particular problems, he will send out certain cues; the nurse is responsible for observing these. Through her observations of cues, she is able to make diagnoses, then to decide on the best course of action to follow for the client's benefit.[56] These authors suggest that nurses have been engaged in this inferential process since the beginning of nursing but that there has not been a critical, deliberate, and systematic analysis of the process until recently. The *lens model* they suggest is easily adapted to the process of nursing. Significant landmarks of the model are: identification of the state of the patient from which cues are read or interpreted, deduction of inferences, and the planning and implementation of action according to defined goals. The authors illustrated the effectiveness of thorough analysis and the potential for study available in the fertile and complex nurse–client encounter.

To narrow the gap between the discovery of new knowledge and its application to the practice of nursing, Imogene King suggested that general concepts be identified; these then form a broad base. As new knowledge is gained, the data acquired can be integrated into concepts already identified. Dr. King is to be saluted for making significant presentations of her own definition of nursing, defining and discussing concepts she believes are fundamental to its practice, and projecting their potential use in the development of a frame of reference that can be used for research in nursing practice. Nursing is defined by King as a process of action, reaction, interaction, and transaction whereby nurses assist individuals of any age group to meet their basic human needs in coping with their health status at some particular point in their life cycle. She suggests five concepts as a basis for organizing knowledge for nursing practice: perception, communication, interpersonal relationships, health, and social institutions.[62, 63]

At present, the term *nursing process* is viewed as the core process by which the purposes of nursing are fulfilled. In addition to nurses who developed concepts of the nursing process as a whole, others have contributed significantly to concepts about elements of the process, such as nursing history,[64, 65] nursing diagnosis,[66, 67] nursing orders and nursing care plans,[68, 69] and nursing evaluation.[70, 71]

Nursing Process

Dividing the process into phases is an artificial separation of actions that in actual practice cannot be separated. To insure a deliberateness and thoughtfulness in analysis of the process, however, it is necessary to label the phases and suggest that the practitioner make a concerted effort to name each action in terms of the phase of nursing she is performing. This practice will insure that the *how* of the nursing process and the *how* of nursing action are carefully, consciously, and deliberately pursued. The *what* of nursing will not be as uniformly labeled as the *how* of nursing, for the *what* will vary with each client. To facilitate the discussion and performance of nursing, the nursing process is divided into the following components or phases: assessing, planning, implementing, and evaluating. Although other authors use similar names for each phase of the process, it is believed that these four labels best identify the phases through which nursing proceeds. Each phase of the nursing process will be defined and the components of each phase will be identified so as to introduce theories basic to the nursing process as presented in Chapter 2. An in-depth analysis and discussion of each of the four phases of the nursing process will be presented in Chapter 3.

Pre-process

To conduct the nursing process, a minimum of two persons is necessary. Usually more than two persons are significant to the client and/or the nurse in each situation. As the number of persons increases in a situation, the complexity of the situation increases. Each individual in the situation brings his unique experiences and attributes to the encounter that is nursing and it is these variables that alter, modify, simplify, or complicate each event experienced in an encounter.

As the nurse prepares to initiate the process of nursing, she considers the status of the client by asking herself questions such as: What experiences does he bring to this situation? What knowledge does he possess and what does he lack: which strengths will help him cope? In what limitations will he be dependent on others?

Initiating the process of nursing requires a consideration of the status of the nurse as well as the client; for example, the nurse asks herself: What approach will be the best to use for this person? How can the nurse most efficiently and effectively set the stage for the provision of nursing? What assistance will the nurse need, and from whom, to best care for this client?

Within this framework of questions the nurse anticipates the initiation of the nursing process and prepares for a productive client–nurse encounter. The tone of the meeting will be established by the degree of interest and trust that can be communicated to the client at the outset of the process. Greeting the client and introducing the nurse are amenities that are expected but sometimes overlooked. Through a deliberate approach to the nursing process the following pre-process goals will be achieved:

1. Establishment of a degree of trust between client and nurse.
2. Definition of the role the nurse will play in the client's care.
3. An opportunity for the client to voice initial fears, raise pressing questions, begin to feel a degree of comfort in the client role.
4. A positive environment in which to permit successful pursuit of the nursing process.

Whether or not the nurse accomplishes these identified goals, prior to the initiation of or within the nursing process itself is not so important as the fact that the accomplishment of the goals is necessary to pursue the nursing process effectively. In some instances pursuit of the pre-process goals enables the process to be initiated with increased ease; in other situations, it is easier to incorporate these pre-process goals within the assessment phase of the nursing process.

Assessing

Assessing is the act of reviewing a situation for the purpose of diagnosing the client's problems.

Just as the total nursing process is a series of systematic, organized, and deliberate acts, so the assessment phase of the process is a series of systematic, organized, and deliberate acts. These actions include examining the client and identifying cues, collecting and analyzing the data, and reaching conclusions.

Examining the Client

Each person for whom the nurse has responsibility is unique and individual. All persons have the same basic human needs, but each person meets his own needs differently. Each person who becomes ill or deviates from his usual, or normal state, attempts to cope with health problems in his own way. It is the challenge presented to the nurse, as she proceeds to examine the client, to determine his problems as he perceives them. What is it that is troubling the client? What is interfering with his usual or normal functioning or his normal coping mechanisms? As the nurse assesses, she engages in the activities of inspection and communication.

Inspection requires the use of hands (touch), eyes (sight), ears (hearing), and nose (smelling), as well as astute judgment, sound decision making, and keen perception. The use of all these skills is crucial to the nurse as she collects data about alterations in the client's physical being, his behavior, and his role or his status in the family and/or society. Use of techniques for physical examination is important in some situations whereas use of techniques for examining behaviors and role change is just as important in others. The challenge faced by the nurse is the development and efficient use of the appropriate skills as dictated by the presenting problems. For example, efficiency in percussion and auscultation techniques may be needed in some situations and not in others. Efficiency in using interviewing skills may be most important in certain situations. It is the nurse's responsibility to determine which skills are to be used, which data are to be collected, and which avenues are to be explored, depending on the client's situation.

Communication with the client is a necessary and continuous activity. The nurse uses communication not only to obtain data, but also to validate with the client the observations she has made. At times different persons perceive the same problem in different ways, so the nurse continually checks to insure that she knows how the client is perceiving the identified problem.

To further enhance the organization and systematic process of assessment, it is wise to use some plan for data collection. For example, a physical assessment can proceed from head to toe to insure consideration of all parts of the body. A body system plan is another framework that can be used. Either of these can be incorporated into a framework such as Maslow's hierarchy,[72] which provides a much broader base for data collection than either a head-to-toe or a body systems plan. Within such a hierarchy, human needs are identified, and through their assessment, the nurse determines in which area of need there is a problem. For example, the first level, the physiologic needs, require assessment of such things as mobility, circulation, nutrition, elimination, air, and oxygen. The next level, safety and security, includes needs such as dependency, protection, freedom from fear, and need for order. Assessment continues up the hierarchy to the highest level of self-actualization. All levels must be kept in mind as client needs are assessed and problems defined.

Collecting and Analyzing the Data

Having examined the client and his situation, the nurse will have collected certain data that are then analyzed. The nurse summarizes the collected data, collates the data, groups together similar data, and arranges the data in some sequence or orderly form so that reasonable conclusions can be drawn. Ingredients for baking a cake have individual characteristics initially but take on different appearances and qualities as they are mixed together and blended with each other. Likewise, each bit of data collected about the client is looked at in relation to the other pieces of data and at how each facet of information is affected by other data in order to attempt to perceive the dimensions of the client situation.

Reaching Conclusions

The final step in the assessment phase of the nursing process is defining the nursing diagnosis; that is, reaching conclusions about the data that have been collected and analyzed.

Nursing diagnoses are defined in various ways, although a review of several definitions reveals certain common elements.

Roy defines nursing diagnosis as a summary statement or a conclusion based on data gathered in the assessment process.[73]

McCain considers it to be an identification of the client's functional disabilities or symptoms, as well as an identification of his most important functional abilities.[74]

Aspinall sees it as a process of clinical inferences from observed changes in a client's physical or psychologic condition.[75]

Gordon defines a diagnostic category with three components, namely, health problem, or state of the client; etiology of the problem; and signs and symptoms of the problem. She refers to this as the PES syndrome—the problem, etiology, and signs/symptoms.[76]

The names of nurses Gebbie and Lavin from St. Louis are now synonymous with the effort to classify nursing diagnoses. They perceive the term nursing diagnosis as a troublesome one for some, but suggest that this should not prevent the establishment of legitimate nursing diagnoses as well as definition of signs and symptoms specific to certain nursing diagnoses.[66] The prescribed nursing interventions to alleviate the problems of the client logically follow the identification of these signs and symptoms.

Discussions among nurses usually identify what a nursing diagnosis is and what it is not, in order to differentiate and relate this term to some of the more familiar jargon and activities in nursing. Nursing diagnosis is identified as the end product of the assessment process; it is a statement of conclusion, either tentative or definitive, drawn by the nurse after having assessed the client's status, that is, after having collected and made some judgment about the data. The nursing diagnosis is an expression of the status of the client with identification of his assets and strengths as well as his disturbances and weaknesses. It is a "statement of a patient problem arrived at by making inferences about the collected data. The problem is one that can be alleviated by nursing intervention." [77]

Nursing diagnosis is not the same as the goals set for the client, nor is the term to be used synonymously with nursing interventions. It forms the basis for setting goals and for planning interventions but it is not the same element as these activities.

Finally, nursing diagnosis is not a medical diagnosis. The nursing diagnosis is a client problem amenable to nursing intervention, whereas a medical diagnosis is a client problem amenable to medical intervention. It will be necessary for a period of time to use the adjectives *nursing* and *medical* with the word diagnosis until both professions become familiar and comfortable with the distinction between the two terms.

From a legal standpoint, a number of jurisdictions are now including the term *nursing diagnosis* in the definition of nursing in the Nurse Practice Acts. In at least one state, the legal definition of nursing states that the professional nurse "diagnoses and treats human responses to actual and potential health problems." [78]

Bernzweig, a member of the New York bar, states: ". . . nursing diagnosis is an established and independent function of the professional nurse and calls for the utmost in intelligent judgment and sensitivity on her part . . . Good nursing diagnosis is one of the keys to the successful practice of nursing and is therefore a skill all nurses should learn." [79]

Planning

Planning is the determination of what can be done to assist the client; it involves setting goals, judging priorities, and designing methods to resolve problems.

Judicious, careful, and deliberate goal-setting is vital to this phase of the nursing process so that the nursing care plan can be developed. When goals are defined, the blueprint is drawn, and methods are identified for the best means to accomplish established goals.

Having collected pertinent data about the client by means of assessment, the nurse continues to validate these data. By communicating with the client to determine whether the perceptions are correct, the nurse will insure that she and the client are at the same point in the planning phase and that both have assessed and perceived his problems in the same way. Long-range, or ultimate goals, as well as short-range, or proximate goals, will be established, within which priorities are set. The most urgent or the ones that should be achieved first are determined before long-range or more distant goals are set. Proximate goals can be compared to wayside stations, in that they can be attained more quickly; they give both the client and the nurse some degree of satisfaction as well as a sense of accomplishment and some assurance that steps toward the ultimate goal are well directed. Both ultimate and proximate goals are kept in sight, and the actions needed to achieve them proceed simultaneously, but each is at a different stage of development at any given time.

The essence of planning includes a deliberate approach to setting precise goals, both ultimate and proximate, continually validating the data obtained by assessing the client's problems, establishing priorities, and making decisions about specific measures to be used to resolve his problems.

By assessing the client's problems deliberately and systematically through knowledgeable perception, observation, and communication, and validating her findings rather than relying on her intuition, the nurse provides qualitative data from which accurate diagnoses can be made and sound planning developed.[80]

Implementation

Implementation is the initiation and completion of the actions necessary to accomplish defined goals.

Thought and preparation were involved in assessing and planning, and decisions were made about actions required to help the client. As she implements these actions, the nurse will be coordinating the activities of various paramedical personnel and functioning cooperatively with members of the health team for the benefit of the client. The exact number of these persons will vary, depending on the setting in which the client is located. Caring for a client at home will involve different kinds of personnel than, for example, caring for that same client in a medical center in which teaching and research are emphasized. In either setting, the nurse will be coping with people who will be interrupting actions, seeking data about the client, and invading the territory of nurse and client, but all of these people will be a vital part of the health scene.

Personnel from various disciplines, functioning on the health team, are acting on behalf of the client; the mere presence of a number of people in the client's environment necessitates the coordination of their activities to make sure that all are directed toward his best interests. Most of the responsibility for coordinating these actions belongs to the nurse. This implies good skills in interpersonal relations and a knowledge of human behavior. Coordinating the various activities successfully so that defined goals are achieved through the action of various people is a challenging task and one that can act as a major motivating force for the professional nurse.

The nursing team consists of levels of personnel with different kinds of preparation as well as different personality traits and abilities. The nurse assumes responsibility for direct client care and for coordinating the efforts of and directing the activities of nursing personnel. The need to know the potential production level of each member of the nursing team, to know the problems and needs of the clients for whom each is responsible, and to match these two qualities to the best of her ability is involved in this responsibility. This is a constant task, a dynamic activity, to which the committed nurse can address herself with good quality results. The skillful application of techniques of interpersonal relations can result in positive and pleasing outcomes for the client as well as satisfaction for personnel.

Implementation is an action-oriented phase of the nursing process in which the nurse is responsible for implementing the nursing care plan that was developed. To be able to coordinate skillfully the activities of health and nursing team members, minister direct client care, and delegate responsibilities for this care to nursing personnel, according to their backgrounds and abilities, are challenges confronting the nurse during this phase. The intellectual, interpersonal, and technical actions employed during the implementation phase are based on the plan for nursing care designed for the individual client according to his assessed problems.

Evaluation

Evaluation is the appraisal of the changes experienced by the client as a result of the actions of the nurse.

To initiate the evaluation phase, the nurse reviews and reflects on the goals set by the original blueprint or nursing care plan devised for the client. When goals have been established, and aims identified at the outset of client care, the nurse and the client are able to determine whether, and to what extent, they have reached their destination. This process of determining just where they are in goal attainment will involve asking a number of questions such as: What were the expected client behaviors? Is there another way to accomplish the same goals for the client with more efficiency or more effectiveness? What changes should, or could, be made? Did the nurse achieve the goals she set out to accomplish? Should some adjustments be made so that these same actions can be more effective? Planning for future actions for this and other clients will be adjusted or altered by this type of constant examination and inquiry.

For many years, the evaluation phase was the most neglected phase of the nursing process. To identify a few of the several reasons for this neglect, the following are cited. The emphasis on the need for objectivity in evaluation seemed to paralyze the nursing profession into a state of inaction. Rather than proceed with a degree of objectivity, and some subjectivity, while continuing to improve evaluation techniques, nurses chose the "do-nothing" way, and little or no progress was made in evaluating client care. Also, there was a paucity of means (instruments or tools) to guide the nurse in the evaluation of client changes, which interfered with evaluation efforts. With no concrete guides to direct evaluation activities, it is understandable that this phase of nursing could be overlooked. It is difficult if not impossible to measure progress without guidelines.

Although there was a gradual increase in concern for evaluation on the part of the nursing profession generally, and sporadic efforts were being reported in the professional literature, there was no unified force behind the profession's efforts to do a more qualitative evaluation of client care. In other words, evaluation was not mandatory, and it was relatively easy to overlook, to be forgotten, or ignored in the face of other pressures and priorities faced by the nurse.

In the fall of 1967, the President's Health Manpower Commission report suggested that professional societies should function as sponsors and supervisors in performing peer review on a local level.[81] Objectivity and impartiality were stressed and assurance of high quality performance was emphasized. Following the circulation of this report in 1967, hospital utilization review groups were established but had little effect on the quality of care, with the major focus on keeping enough beds available for admissions.

Awareness of the cost escalation of in-patient health services and the large sums being spent on recipients of federal health care resulted in congressional restraints by means of professional controls. These controls were defined in Social Security Amendment P.H.92–603 and became effective in October, 1972.[82] The law is known as the Professional Standards Review Organization Law (PSRO) and mandates that fellow professionals review their peers' actions. Physicians' organizations have priority in establishing PSROs, but nursing services are subject to review as well. Reviews of client care are based on criteria that have been developed by the peer group.

Although nurses are not specifically named in the PSRO law, they are becoming active participants in these review groups because of the legal requirement for peer review and because nursing performance is being reviewed.

The outcome of the PSRO law is an increased awareness of quality care and quality assurance. Emphasis on the rights of clients and the demand for services commensurate with the cost to the client have also contributed to this demand for quality. The following provide evidence of this change in emphasis: The ANA initiated an effort to define nursing standards prior to the PSRO law; standards of care have now been established by the ANA via the Congress for Nursing Practice as models for nursing.[83] Input from all professional nurses is necessary to insure that the adopted standards will continue to reflect the optimum level of care.

Record-keeping has been revised to enable better client care as well as better care review; the revised recording system is known as the Problem-Oriented Medical Record (POMR).[84] Although a variety of approaches is being used, the intent is to focus on the problems encountered by the client and to enable various disciplines associated with the client to systematically record data about his problems.

The use of the SOAP acronym is frequently seen in the POMR system. The collection of subjective data (S) and objective data (O) about the client's problems is a legitimate manner of assessing (A) client's needs in order to plan his care (P). Persons using the SOAPIER acronym are pursuing nursing more completely, however; adding "IER" insures the implementation (I) and evaluation (E) phases of care and provides for the reassessment (R) of client's needs when that is necessary.

Outcome criteria are being defined [85] with increasing frequency, and mutual goals are being set by the client and the nurse; in this way, both know the direction and the purpose of care. A review of progress or lack of progress becomes possible when there is a criterion statement against which the care can be measured.

While evaluation of care was a neglected aspect of care in the past, an increasing number of evaluation efforts are being reported in the professional nursing literature. A commendable study was conducted through the efforts of the Nursing Research Branch, Division of Nursing of the National Institute of Health and the Rush-Presbyterian-St. Luke's Medical Center and is reported in two parts: Part I presents a method for monitoring quality of nursing care in hospitals,[86] and Part II reports the testing of the methodology to examine the components of quality as well as outcomes of care.[87]

As a result of the first phase of this study, a methodology was developed for evaluating the quality of care in medical, surgical, pediatric, and related intensive care units. The framework for the evaluation was based on six major objectives within which a master list of criteria was developed that formed the basis for the monitoring of care. A review of the master list of criteria reveals a comprehensive coverage of all aspects of care with a nursing process orientation. Extensive data are included in the area of assessment; basic human needs are considered in their entirety so that assessment of the needs of clients is complete if the master list is used. A good balance is maintained in specifying physical and nonphysical needs; the nonphysical needs are identified as psychologic, emotional, mental, social, and spiritual. Included in the monitoring process are the patient's family, the other personnel in the hospital, such as administrators and managers, the environment in which the client finds himself in the hospital, and the record-keeping system.

Stated implications for nursing were derived from this well-organized and carefully conducted study. One of the highlights is the fact that the nursing process emphasis ". . . is not only appropriate and desirable but also necessary for meeting the goal of maximum effectiveness of care." [88] The recommendations for future studies as stated by the directors of this project are pertinent and challenging. Basic to all suggestions for the future, however, is a firm grasp of the nursing process in all of its dimensions.

Tucker et al. have published a guideline for the nurse to use in caring for clients entitled *Patient Care Standards.*[89] It is suggested that these standards will be useful in planning care, in defining outcome criteria, and in auditing the quality of the care given.

Phaneuf's efforts in nursing audit predate the mandatory PSRO groups.[90] In the second edition of *The Nursing Audit,* Phaneuf suggests concrete guides to persons concerned with quality control in a variety of patient care settings.[91] She clarifies terms, presents examples of instruments for use in auditing and provides direction for implementation of the auditing activity.

Two additional publications are advantageous in performing an evaluation of client care. *The Slater Nursing Competency Rating Scale* is intended to measure the nurse's competencies.[92] This is a retrospective instrument and can be used in any setting where nurses engage in various nurse–client interactions.

Wandelt and Ager developed a *Quality Patient Care Scale* (QUALPACS), which is intended to measure care received by the client.[93] It is derived from the Slater Scale and in many instances the items on both scales are the same except for the wording of an item. Qualpacs focuses on the care received by the client and the Slater Scale focuses on how the care was performed by the nurse.

From a more quiescent state, therefore, it appears that evaluation of client care is assuming importance in the pursuit of nursing. With further attention to evaluation by all disciplines concerned with health maintenance and care during illness, and especially attention to all facets of evaluation by the professional nurse group, clients will benefit from increasingly improved care.

Summary

The profession of nursing has moved through a number of developmental stages that can be relatively well-defined by reflecting on the progress of nursing through the years. From debating about whether or not nursing is a profession, the group has moved to the more serious concern of defining the essence of nursing. A number of authors have suggested ideas and definitions that identify the unique nature of nursing according to individual orientations and philosophies. Concepts of nursing are being identified with increasing frequency, and more precise and qualifying theories are emerging. Eventually, the science of nursing will be clearly defined. Finally, the nursing process is being viewed as the very core of nursing, and although there are several ways by which each phase or component of the process is labeled, the idea of the process is recognized and the steps through which the nurse proceeds to effect client care have the general support of nursing.

References

1. Frank CM: Foundations of Nursing. Philadelphia, Saunders, 1959, p 78
2. Nightingale F: Notes on Nursing. What It Is and What It Is Not. (facsimile of 1859 edition). Philadelphia, Lippincott, 1946
3. Brown EL: Nursing For the Future. New York, Russell Sage Foundation, 1948
4. Flexner A: Universities. New York, Oxford University Press, 1930, pp 29–31
5. Schein EH: Professional Education—Some New Directions. New York, McGraw-Hill, 1972, pp 7–14
6. Coladarci AP: What about that word profession? Am J Nurs 63:116–118, October 1963
7. Code for Nurses. *The American Nurse,* Kansas City, Mo., October 15, 1976, p 5
8. American Nurses' Association's First Position on Education For Nursing. Am J Nurs 65:106–111, December 1965
9. Nayer DD: The ANA position paper. Imprint 23:23ff, February 1976
10. US Department of Health, Education, and Welfare, Public Health Service. Toward Quality in Nursing. Needs and Goals. Report of the Surgeon General's Consultant Group in Nursing. Washington, DC: US Government Printing Office, 1963
11. Lysaught JP: An Abstract For Action. New York, McGraw-Hill, 1970, pp 81–147
12. Mauksch IG, Young PR: Nurse–physician interaction in a family medical care center. Nurs Outlook 22:113–119, February 1974
13. Kinlein ML: Independent nurse practitioner. Nurs Outlook 20:22–24, January 1972
14. Two New York nurses debate the NYSNA 1985 proposal. Am J Nurs 76:930–935, June 1976
15. ANA Convention '76. Am J Nurs 76:1127, July 1976
16. Study of credentialing launched. Am J Nurs 76:1893–1895, December 1976
17. Ozimek D, Yura H: Who is the Nurse Practitioner? New York, National League for Nursing, 1975

18. Bloch D: Some crucial terms in nursing—what do they really mean? Nurs Outlook 22:689–694, November 1974
19. Gowan MO: Administration of college and university programs in nursing, from the viewpoint of nurse education. Proceedings of the Workshop on Administration of College Programs in Nursing. Washington, DC, The Catholic University of America Press, 1944, p 10
20. Kreuter FR: What is good nursing care? Nurs Outlook 5:302–304, May 1957
21. Erikson EH: Childhood and Society, second edition. New York, Norton, 1963, pp 247–251
22. Johnson DE: A philosophy of nursing. Nurs Outlook 7:198–200, April 1959
23. ———: The nature of a science of nursing. Nurs Outlook 7:291–294, May 1959
24. Wiedenbach E: The helping art of nursing. Am J Nurs 63:54–57, 1963
25. Henderson V: The Nature of Nursing. New York, Macmillan, 1966, p 15
26. Norris CM: Delusions that trap nurses. Nurs Outlook 21:18–21, January 1973
27. *Ibid,* p 21
28. McAllister JB: A Syllabus of Logic. Washington, DC, The Catholic University of America, 1942, p 15
29. Dickoff J, James P: Beliefs and values: bases for curriculum design. Nurs Res 19:415, September–October 1970
30. Jacox A: Theory construction in nursing: an overview. Nurs Res 23:4–13, January–February 1974
31. Webster's Third International Dictionary. Springfield, Mass., Merriam, 1967
32. Torres G, Yura H: *Today's Conceptual Framework: Its Relationship to the Curriculum Development Process.* New York, National League for Nursing, 1974, p 2
33. Johnson MM, Martin HW: A sociological analysis of the nurse role. Am J Nurs 58:373–377, March 1958
34. McKay RP: The Process of Theory Development in Nursing. New York, Teachers College, Columbia University, A Report of an Ed D Project, 1965, p 16
35. Horgan MV: Concepts about Nursing in Selected Nursing Literature from 1950–1965. Unpublished Masters Dissertation, The Catholic University of America, School of Nursing, Washington DC, 1967
36. Dickoff J, James P, Wiedenbach E: Theory in a practice discipline, Part II. Practice oriented research, Nurs Res 17:552, November–December 1968
37. King IM: Toward a Theory of Nursing. New York, Wiley, 1971, chap 2, pp 10–30
38. Orem DE: Nursing: Concepts of Practice. New York, McGraw-Hill, 1971

39. Nursing Development Conference Group: Concept Formalization in Nursing—Process and Product. Boston, Little, Brown, 1973
40. Riehl JP, Roy C: Conceptual Models for Nursing Practice. New York, Appleton-Century-Crofts, 1974
41. Rogers ME: Nursing Science: An Introduction to the Theoretical Basis of Nursing. Philadelphia, Davis, 1970
42. Roy C: Introduction to Nursing: An Adaptation Model. New Jersey, Prentice-Hall, 1976
43. Travelbee J: Interpersonal Aspects of Nursing, second edition, Philadelphia, Davis, 1971
44. Zderad L, Belcher H: Developing Behavioral Concepts in Nursing. Atlanta, Southern Regional Educational Board, 1968
45. Hardy ME (ed): Theoretical Foundations for Nursing. New York, MSS Information Corporation, 1973
46. Bevis EO: Curriculum Building in Nursing—A Process. St. Louis, Mosby, 1973, p 9
47. Yura H, Ozimek, D, Walsh MB: Nursing Leadership: Theory and Process. New York, Appleton-Century-Crofts, 1976, p 95
48. Wandelt MA: Guide for the Beginning Researcher. New York, Appleton-Century-Crofts, 1970, p xvii
49. McDonald FJ, Harms MT: A theoretical model for an experimental curriculum. Nurs Outlook 14:48–50, August 1966
50. Hall LE: Quality of Nursing Care. Address at meeting of Department of Baccalaureate and Higher Degree Programs of the New Jersey League for Nursing, February 7, 1955, Seton Hall University, Newark, New Jersey. Published in Public Health News, New Jersey State Department of Health, June, 1955
51. Orlando IJ: The Dynamic Nurse-Patient Relationship. New York, Putnam's, 1961, p 26
52. Knowles LN: Decision making in nursing—a necessity for doing, ANA Clinical Sessions, 1966. New York, Appleton-Century-Crofts, 1967, pp 248–272
53. Defining Clinical Content, Graduate Nursing Programs, Medical and Surgical Nursing. Boulder, Colorado, Western Interstate Commission on Higher Education, 1967, p 6
54. Yura H, Walsh MB (eds): The Nursing Process, first edition, Washington DC, The Catholic University of America Press, 1967
55. Kelly KJ: An approach to the study of clinical inference in nursing. Nurs Res 13:314–322, fall 1964
56. ———: Clinical inference in nursing—a nurse's viewpoint. Nurs Res 15:23–26, winter 1966
57. Hammond KR: Clinical inference in nursing—a psychologist's viewpoint. Nurs Res 15:27–38, winter 1966
58. Hammond KR, Kelly KJ, Schneider RJ, Vancini M: Clinical inference in nursing-analyzing cognitive tasks representative of nursing problems. Nurs Res 15:134–138, spring 1966

59. ———: Clinical inference in nursing-information units used. Nurs Res 15:236–243, summer 1966
60. Hammond KR, Kelly KJ, Castellan NJ Jr, Schneider RJ, Vancini M: Clinical inference in nursing: use of information-seeking strategies. Nurs Res 15:330–336, fall 1966
61. Hammond KR, Kelly KJ, Schneider RJ, Vancini M: Clinical inference in nursing: revising judgments. Nurs Res 16:38–45, winter 1967
62. King IM: A conceptual frame of reference for nursing. Nurs Res 17:27–31, 1968
63. ———: Toward a Theory for Nursing. New York, Wiley, 1971
64. McPhetridge LM: Nursing History: One means to personalized care. Am J Nurs 68:68–75, January 1968
65. Becknell EP, Smith DM: System of Nursing Practice. Philadelphia, Davis, 1975
66. Gebbie K, Lavin MA: Classifying Nursing Diagnoses. Am J Nurs 74:250–253, February 1974
67. Gordon M: Nursing diagnosis and the diagnostic process. Am J Nurs 76:1298–1300, August 1976
68. Little DE, Carnevali DL: Nursing Care Planning, 2nd edition. Philadelphia, Lippincott, 1976
69. Mayers MG: A Systematic Approach to the Nursing Care Plan. New York, Appleton-Century-Crofts, 1972
70. Phaneuf MC: The Nursing Audit, second edition. New York, Appleton-Century-Crofts, 1976
71. Wandelt MA, Stewart DS: Slater Nursing Competencies Rating Scale. New York, Appleton-Century-Crofts, 1975.
72. Maslow AH: Motivation and Personality, second edition, New York, Harper & Row, 1970, pp 35–46
73. Roy C: A diagnostic classification system for nursing. Nurs Outlook 23:90–94, February 1975
74. McCain F: Nursing by assessment, not intuition. Am J Nurs 65:82–85, April 1965
75. Aspinall MJ: Nursing diagnosis—the weak link. Nurs Outlook 24:433–436 July 1976
76. Gordon M: Nursing diagnoses and the diagnostic process. Am J Nurs 76:1298–1300, August 1976
77. Mundinger MO, Jauron GD: Developing a nursing diagnosis. Nurs Outlook 23:96, February 1975
78. *Ibid,* p 94
79. Gebbie KM, Lavin MA: Classification of Nursing Diagnoses. St. Louis, Mosby, 1975, pp 28–29
80. McCain F: Nursing by assessment, not intuition. Am J Nurs 65:82–84, April 1965
81. Wilson R: PSRO's in nursing: what are they? Imprint 23:36–37, April 1976
82. Public Law 92–603, 92nd Congress, HRI, October 30, 1972

83. Standards of Nursing Practice. Kansas City, American Nurses' Association, 1973
84. Weed LL: Medical records that guide and teach. New Engl J Med 278:598–599, March 14, 1968
85. Berg H: Nursing audit and outcome criteria. Nurs Clin NA, 9:331–335, June 1974
86. Jelinek, RC, et al: A Methodology for Monitoring Quality of Nursing Care. Bethesda, Md.: US Department of Health, Education, and Welfare, 1974
87. Haussmann RKD, et al: Monitoring Quality of Nursing Care. Bethesda, Md.: US Department of Health, Education, and Welfare, 1976
88. *Ibid,* p 65
89. Tucker SM, et al: Patient Care Standards. St. Louis, Mosby, 1975
90. Phaneuf MC: The Nursing Audit—Profile for Excellence. New York, Appleton-Century-Crofts, 1972
91. Phaneuf MC: The Nursing Audit—Self-Regulation in Nursing Practice. New York, Appleton-Century-Crofts, 1976
92. Wandelt MA, Stewart DS: Slater Nursing Competencies Rating Scale. New York, Appleton-Century-Crofts, 1975
93. Wandelt MA, Ager JW: Quality Patient Care Scale. New York, Appleton-Century-Crofts, 1974

Chapter Two •

Theoretical Framework for the Nursing Process

The nursing process is a designated series of actions intended to fulfill the purposes of nursing—to maintain the client's wellness—and, if this state changes, to provide the amount and quality of nursing care his situation demands to direct him back to wellness, and if wellness cannot be achieved, to contribute to his quality of life, maximizing his resources as long as life is a reality. Inherent in these purposes is the fulfillment and maintenance of the integrity of the human needs of the person. To fulfill these purposes, the development of the idea of the nursing process and the beginning development of its theoretical framework must be considered.

Many different theories from various disciplines suggest a relationship to the nursing process. These include general systems theory, information theory, communication theory, decision and problem-solving theories, theories of perception and human need theories. General systems theory seems to be applicable in a broad way. Information, communication, decision, and problem-solving theories stem from general systems theory and give support in a more specific manner. Selections from these theories give credence to the nurse's as well as the client's actions, with these and human need theory providing a framework within which the nursing process can be analyzed and applied.

General Systems Theory

General systems theory provides a framework for dealing with complex problems and the changing relationships inherent within and among them. A system can be viewed as an entity composed of interrelated interacting parts or components. A system is comprised of purpose, process, and content. Purpose refers to that which must be accomplished and therefore gives direction to the system; content refers to the parts that make up the system, and the process of the system and its operations are functions of the parts in fulfilling the purpose for which the system was developed. Banathy states that the best way to identify a system is to reveal its purpose.[1]

General systems theory took hold in the post-World War II years; it was introduced as early as 1937 by Ludwig von Bertalanffy when it appeared that there were laws within this system that applied to all systems of a certain type, irrespective of their particular properties and the elements involved. Thus, von Bertalanffy postulated a general system theory whose subject matter is the result of a formulation of principles valid for all systems, regardless of the nature of or the relationship between their component elements. The aim of general systems theory is to integrate the various fields of science with unifying principles that extend vertically through each individual science.[2] Thus, communication between specialists from different disciplines could be enhanced, and the duplication of effort resulting from identical formulations developed independently could be eliminated. General systems theory provides the structure through which a whole may be divided into its component parts so that the relationship or force between them can be studied and manipulated. It also provides a structure whereby unconnected parts may be integrated into an organized whole.

A system may be composed of subsystems, each designed to carry out a purpose, which, in turn, is necessary in achieving the general purpose of the system. Nursing operates within the context of the health care system and, as such, may be considered one of its subsystems. The health care system is not an enclosed self-sustaining one but one that operates within the environment that gives it its purpose. Society can be considered the suprasystem of the health care system, for the former gives the latter its purpose. Thus, the health care system has its own purpose, process, and content, as well as its own resources, demands, and limitations. Many other systems—educational, political, industrial—operate within the suprasystem of society. The health care system operates cooperatively in conjunction with these other systems. Within the health care system there are a number of subsystems designed to carry out the purpose of the health care system. Nursing, medicine, dentistry, and pharmacy are but a few of such subsystems. Each carries out a specific purpose which, in turn, contributes to attaining that of the health care system. Subsystems that operate in an integrated cooperative manner contribute to the effectiveness of the health care system, thus fulfilling the purpose for which it exists, as designated by society. The health care system derives input from the suprasystem—society. Through interacting components (functioning within their purposes, input, and resources as derived from the suprasystem), output is produced and fed back into the suprasystem. The closer the output satisfies the purpose for which the system exists, the more acceptable the output will be to the suprasystem. Society will reject output that does not fulfill its purpose. Therefore, the system's output must be assessed continually to make sure that it is adequate. Effective feedback from the suprasystem is needed to maintain its compatibility and viability, which implies a sensitivity to the changing needs and purposes of society and a willingness to make appropriate adjustments. The system will need to look into itself for ways of maximizing the interaction of its components, as well as to assess the effectiveness with which each subsystem within the health care system is performing.[3] The diagram in Figure 1 incorporates the system idea.

With nursing considered a subsystem of the health care system, general systems theory can provide a useful framework for the study of nursing. The concepts and principles of general systems theory offer a decision-making structure as well as a set of strategies that could be used to arrive at a decision. These comprise a self-correcting logical process for assessing, planning, implementing, and evaluating a plan of action to fulfill the purposes of nursing. Basically, this is a practical application of the problem-solving method. Figure 2 demonstrates the interacting elements of the nursing subsystem—the nurse and the client. Nurse and client are each unique in that they have different behavior systems. Thus, the dynamic interaction between the behavior of the nurse and

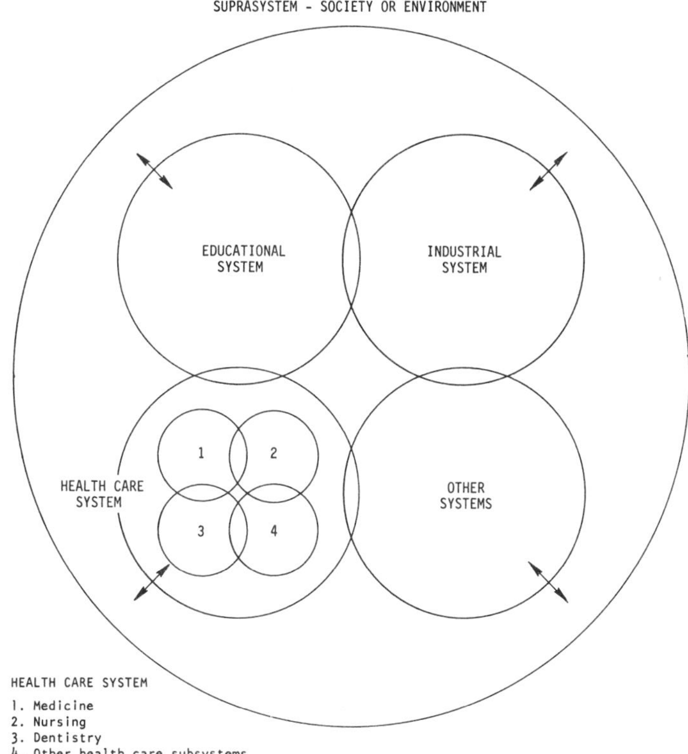

Figure 1.

that of the person or persons who are the client(s) constitute a complex organized whole. The nursing process, with its components—assessing, planning, implementing, and evaluating—constitutes a unifying process utilized to fulfill the purposes of nursing. By means of the nursing process information is processed, problems are designated, alternatives for action are delineated, and a selection is made for implementation. Evaluation is built into the process, with the important aspects of reassessment and modification to insure the purposefulness of acts directed toward a specified goal. Influencing factors related to nursing that have an impact on elements of the system include role designations, role expectations, educational preparation and level, place of interaction, history and tradition, trends, economy, values, transportation, and availability of health services.

The concepts pertaining to general systems theory are open

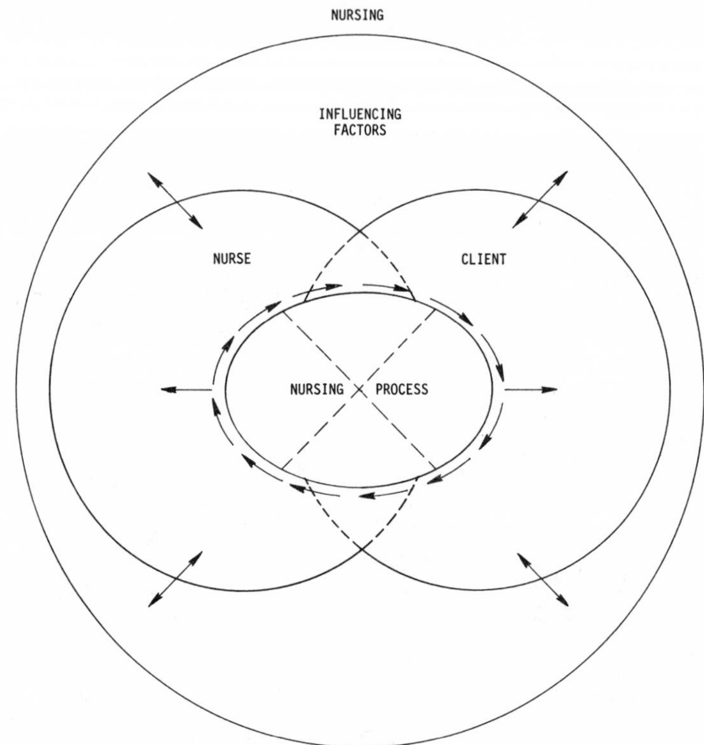

Figure 2.

systems, closed systems, energy and matter, entropy, negentropy, information, and feedback. Systems may be closed or open. A closed system is considered isolated from its environment in that matter, energy, or information are not exchanged with it. Laws of thermodynamics focus only on closed systems. In these systems a certain quantity must increase to a maximum and the process eventually stops in a state of equilibrium. The resulting certain quantity is called entropy, and in a closed system the tendency is toward maximum entropy or disorder. Thus, a system is closed if no material leaves or enters it.

The open system is one in which there is an exchange of matter, energy, or information with the environment. A person is viewed as a living behaving system. The nurse and the client can each be studied as a person. For example, let us consider the biochemical, psychosocial, value, and attitudinal systems of each person. Each of these systems are subsystems; each has its own purpose which, in turn, contributes to the functioning of a person as a whole as well as to the goals of that person. In nursing, the nurse and the client interact in a dynamic fashion for a purpose.

An open system maintains itself in a continuous inflow and outflow, building up its components and breaking them down, but never reaching a state of equilibrium. The open system maintains itself in a steady state. The composition of the system remains constant despite the fact that energy, matter, or information are imported and exported; the process is one of building up and breaking down, in spite of continuous irreversible processes. There are remarkable regulatory characteristics evident in the steady state. This steadiness is referred to as the principle of equifinality. A steady state can be reached from different initial conditions and after disturbances develop in the process.[4] A living system can avoid an increase in entropy and develop toward a state of increased order and organization.[5] An example of this type of exchange is the temperature regulating system of the body,[6] wherein the body increases the amount of heat it produces when it enters a cool environment. Shivering is one method whereby the body increases its heat production and a person may add to it by putting on more clothing or turning up the thermostat. A hot environment induces a response designed to cool the body—sweating. The evaporation of moisture on the surface of the skin has a cooling effect. Additional measures might include removing some clothing, lowering the temperature setting of a thermostat, or turning on an air conditioner. The metabolic, the growth, and the total processes of living and being involve the interchange of energy, matter, or information among parts of the living organism and between the living organism and its environment. The energy or information that is taken in or absorbed is called input; the energy, matter, or information that passes out of the organism into the environment is called output.[7] When viewed solely as a behaving system, man is quite simple. However, the complex environment in which man exists is reflected in the obvious complexity of man's behavior as it develops with age. Hazzard points out that the living organism is an excellent example of a system, because it comprises many interrelated elements and is capable of developing toward states of increased order, organization, differentiation, or disintegration.[8]

Energy and matter are additional concepts pertaining to general systems theory. Energy, in a physical sense, means the capacity to do work and overcome resistance. Matter can be defined as a space-occupying mass—the substance that can be exchanged.

Entropy can be used as an indication of the state of health of a living system. Raymond believes that life processes that are disturbed because matter or energy is poorly transmitted through the organism may, at times, be viewed in terms of deficiencies in information for the direction of required reactions. As the structural and behavioral information content of various parts of the body is destroyed, entropy increases as the living system proceeds toward death. The degenerative processes of nature are balanced when the steady state is maintained by fuels that have a high free-energy content and by communicated information. In the person, communication is carried on through the nervous system, by the transmission of pressure through the vascular system, and through the production and transport of hormones and enzymes. The living system needs sufficient information to facilitate rapid adjustment to a wide variety of information inputs so that growth and adaptability will be enhanced.[9] The human organism's struggle to grow and to develop is accomplished by a continual interchange of matter, energy, or information between it and the environment. The goal is a steady state, maximizing negative entropy as the human organism tends to approach order.

The nurse and the client are regarded as a system that has a certain repertoire of internal and external basic acts, various combinations and sequences of which make up its behaviors. The client may be an individual or a family. A family fulfills the criteria defining a system because it consists of interrelated parts that are capable of reacting to changes in the environment in its efforts to maintain a steady state. If the behavior of the human organism is directed toward adapting to its environment, the selective process by which its basic acts are linked together must be organized according to the current status of the environment relative to the organism.[10]

The ideas of information and feedback provide a frame of reference for viewing a wide range of situations. The person is viewed as a living, behaving system and as an open system engaged in dynamic interchange with his environment. He is self-organizing, adaptive, self-aware, goal-seeking, and he learns. He needs information and depends on the process of communication between and/or among systems as well as subsystems and their environments.[11] Information is defined as some type of event in the physical world that will permit movement over space.[12] Rapaport defines a quantity of information as a signal selected from a set or matched with an element of a set.[13]

Information in the context of general systems theory is measured in terms of decisions and selective process. Information is similar to negative entropy, which is a measure of order. The concept of information is viewed as a tool for quantifying data; that of entropy and negative entropy or negentropy refers to the measure of order and disorder in a system. Entropy is recognized as a measure of disorder. Schrödinger states that every happening, event, and process occurring in nature means that in that part of the world where they are occurring entropy has increased. A living organism continually increases its entropy, tending to approach the dangerous state of maximum entropy–death. Feeding on negative entropy by eating, breathing, drinking, and assimilating, the living organism avoids death.[14]

Feedback is a process whereby information about output from a system is communicated back to that system so that it can be evaluated and regulated. It constitutes the control mechanism of the system, relating output back to its source so that it is possible to make adjustments, adaptations, and modifications. Feedback is an extremely important component if the system is to regulate itself. The evaluation component of the nursing process incorporates feedback in designating a problem-solution or a need for reassessment.

Information and Communication Theories

In addition to the theoretical framework provided by general systems theory in a broad sense, additional theoretical formulations relating to information and communication, decision and problem-solving, and perception provide more insight into the basis for these processes. These theories have contributed to systems theory. A cardinal feature of information theory is that it is a theory of selection–selection from well-defined sets of alternatives. To make a selection is to make a decision. Such a theory is statistical in the sense that probability must be considered.[15] The wider the choice is, the larger is the set of alternatives open to use. The more uncertain one is about how to proceed, the more information that person requires before he can make a decision. A component of efficient communication is the analysis of how a person selects and codes available stimuli, that is, how effectively he processes his input. Information and communication theories focus on the fundamental nature of the mediating linkage underlying the interrelations and interactions of the parts that comprise a complex living, behaving system. A person needs information when confronted with a choice to make. Information processes, being selective, demand that selections be made from a set of alternatives. If the sequence of selection is to convey information, the possible choice must be known to the person who is to receive that information. It is necessary to consider the choices available to us and the probabilities associated with each.[16] The information transmitted depends on the manner and effectiveness of processing and organizing sensory input from the environment. Information is the number of potential choices provided from which effective courses of action can be selected. Ackoff states that to inform is to provide a basis for choice–a belief in the greater efficiency of one choice over another. He believes that information modifies the objective probabilities of choice by modifying subjective estimates of probabilities of success. Instruction is seen as modifying the probabilities of success. Further, a person's state of instruction can be characterized by the amount of control he can exercise over the outcomes within his sphere of responsibility. The more capable a person is in bringing about any of the outcomes possible, the greater control he has over that outcome. This capability can be acquired through instruction.[17]

Communication focuses on the essential nature of the mediating connection underlying the interrelations and interactions within and between systems. The concept of meaning is included in the discussion of communication because both the sender and receiver must know what a given set of symbols signifies. The components of a communication system are source, transmitter, channel, receiver, and destination. The source formulates meaning into a message and the transmitter encodes or transforms that message into information. The source and transmitter are different phases of the act of communication initiated by the person who originated or sent the message. The channel for transmission may be the atmosphere, in the case of a verbal message. If it is written, telegraphic or other means are used to carry the information from one area to another.[18] The receiver decodes the information by transforming its physical aspects into a message. Transformation into the final component, "destination," whose function is to interpret the meaning of the message, is accomplished by means of a person's perceptual abilities. Communication takes place if its meaning at the source of origin coincides with that at its destination. Perfect correspondence between denotative and connotative responses of source and destination is seldom achieved because of interference, which may be mechanical, psychologic, or cultural. This interference, from whatever cause, is called *noise* and needs to be recognized as an additional component of the theoretical system of the act of communication. Correspondence between elements of the response pattern, constituting the meaning at the source and its counterpart at the destination, is reduced, to some degree, by noise.

Another factor in the act of communicating is feedback. The destination operates as a source of feedback, which constitutes a kind of message returning to the communicator. This feedback may take the form of nonverbal communication, and as such can be affected by noise in that gestures or facial expressions can be misunderstood. Thus, this two-way set of components operates as a communication system, with information moving first one way and then another, or in both directions at the same time.[19] This is especially true for person-to-person communication within a system or with persons in other systems. Verbal messages are not the only source of information. A person may also obtain information by observation.

In his informational analysis of responses to questions, Mackay states that a question is basically a purported indication of inadequacy as to the state of readiness of its originator and is calculated to elicit some organizing work to remedy this inadequacy. It would seem that the questioner uncovers and holds out the incomplete portion of his organizing system to the person receiving his attention. Mackay points out that the primary purpose of a question is to update the questioner's own state of readiness. In turn, the meaning of the answer will be its selective function on the range of the questioner's state of orientation.[20]

Ackoff conceptualizes information as relating to the problems the recipient has in reaching a decision. He acknowledges behavioral elements in purposeful states as an individual's objectives, his valuation of each objective, his possible course of action, the efficiency of each course of action in achieving each objective, and his probability of choice for each course of action. The amount of information in a purposeful state is seen in terms of the probabilities of choices for available courses of action, whereas the amount of information in a message is the difference between that following and that preceding the message. Motivation relates to the values the person has placed on the objectives.[21] Communication that changes the probabilities of choice informs. If changes in the efficiency of courses of action are noted, then the communication is one that instructs. When the values of outcome are changed, communication motivates. A single communication may combine information with instruction and motivation.[22] It must be remembered that an inner environment of the living system places limits on the kind of information processing of which the organism is capable of performing. The inner environment imposes very broad limits on organization. Limits are imposed not only on language but also on all other modes of communication, representing, internally, the experiences received through stimuli from outside.[23]

The conceptual framework of information and communication theories can serve as a basis for decision and problem-solving theories, which are seen as the selection and application of a criterion that should be used in selecting a course of action, a purposeful state. Decision theory is concerned with efficiency, value, and effectiveness. Problem-solving theory is concerned with problem determination and resolution.

The purpose of nursing is to identify the client's problems, whether he is well or ill. The nursing process, as the significant process used by the nurse, is basically a decision and problem-solving process. The deliberate use of the nursing process demands that the nurse have knowledge. It involves seeking, selecting, and processing information, judging that information, designating priorities about the information, being aware of alternative courses of action and choosing them, as well as implementing a formulated plan of action. Continuous feedback or evaluation requires appropriate modification of the plan of action to maintain its purposefulness—problem resolution and maintenance of optional wellness. Keen perception, communication, and effective decisions are inherent in this process. The nursing process is cyclic because the need for modification demands reassessment, replanning, renewed implementation, and reevaluation.

Decision and Problem-Solving Theories

Almost every conscious and voluntary movement performed by a person involves a decision of choice. A person's day begins by deciding what time to awake, what to do, to eat, to wear, when and where to sleep, or to do none of these. To make no decision requires a decision. Problem solving is inherent in our day's work and it, too, is filled with decisions. Not only will questions of where, when, and what need to be answered, but the questions of how and for what purpose must also be asked and answered if our immediate, intermediate, and long-range goals as persons are to be realized.

A problem is a question presented for answer or solution. Daniel

Griffiths analyzes the decision-making process within a problem framework and contends that all decision makers operate within a set of limits, thereby improving the caliber of the decisions they make.[24] Preparation for a particular decision begins with the past experiences of the person who is making that decision, before the first formal step is taken in the process.

Within the limitations defined by purpose, the criterion of rationality, conditions of employment, lines of formal authority, relevant information provided, and time limits, the means of arriving at a decision as well as the content of that decision can be prescribed.[25] Wayne Lee described the rationality of decision theory by listing some of the properties of a rational decision. First, he defined the rational person as one who understands his own motivation, then expanded on this to define the rational person (from the standpoint of decision theory) as one who makes a choice (decision) that is best for him when he is confronted with a situation requiring a decision. A rational decision has four properties: (1) it is one or more of a specified set of possible decisions, which is the optimal decision; (2) it depends on the decision principle or rule specifying which set of possible decisions employed by the decision maker is rational or optimal; (3) the rational decision for a situation may differ among persons based on its value or utility to the person, the attractiveness of the consequence, and the impact of this consequence on the decision maker's welfare; and (4) a rational decision is dependent on relevant information available to the person making the decision.[26] According to Lee, "Rationality has been judged only in terms of the choices made, not in terms of the emotional commitment to the choice." [27] While rationality of the decision is viewed in terms of the best or optimal decision, this best decision must be one that is consistent with the decision maker's preferences and beliefs. Lee states, "A person's decision may be rational in one decision situation and nonrational in another. Decisions should be classified according to degree of rationality rather than if rational or not." [28]

The following steps comprise the decision-making process related to a problem situation as outlined by Griffiths: [29]

1. Recognize, define, and limit the problem. The problem becomes known, is delineated, and is stated in terms of either the decision maker's or the client's goal. The problem is stated in a way such that the decision maker can grasp the significance.
2. Analyze the problem. What does the problem mean to the

decision maker and what does it mean to her client? At this point a decision is made as to whether or not a decision should be made.

3. Establish criteria or standards by which a solution will be evaluated or judged as acceptable and adequate to the need. Criteria for evaluation are crucial, and at this stage the value system and aspirations of the individuals involved are built into the process. A decision on criteria and standards must be made prior to the major decision, indicating the sequential nature of the decision-making process.
4. Collect data, more than are necessary. These should be relevant and reproducible.
5. Formulate and select the preferred solution or solutions. Test them in advance. All that has occurred before culminates in a decision—i.e., formulating several solutions, weighing the consequences of each, and selecting a single solution as the one most likely to succeed. The consequences of each solution are weighed and the success of each is predicted by the decision maker, based on his or her knowledge of the probability of the success of the solutions.
6. The preferred solution is put into effect. This involves not only implementing but also modifying the decision as it becomes operational. Subdecisions have been made in each of the preceding steps, and this step is the sequential outcome of other decisions made during the process.[29]

Raiffa focuses on decision analysis under conditions of uncertainty (a state prevalent in nursing situations). In his outline he states that initially the decision maker should list the viable options available for gathering information, for experimentation, and for action. He should then list the events that may possibly occur, arranging the information acquired and the choices made in chronological order. Next, the decision maker determines the acceptability of the consequences that result from the various options for courses of action and judges the chances of the occurrence of any particular uncertain event.[30] These data are used as background for the next steps, which involve a synthesis of information.

The decision maker as a person is viewed as influential in the decision analysis process because of the impact of basic preferences for consequences, judgments about uncertain quantities, and personal understanding of the structure of the decision situation. The achievement of the optimal solution is more likely if the decision maker uses reason and acts in a systematic manner regarding "how an individual who is faced with a problem of choice under uncertainty should go about choosing a course of action that is consistent with his personal basic judgment and preferences. He must consciously police the consistency of his subjective inputs and *calculate* their implications for action." [31]

Raiffa recommends that preferences for consequences be numerically scaled in terms of *utility values* and that judgments about uncertainties be numerically scaled according to probabilities. The concepts of utility and subjective probability are intertwined in the process of decision analysis.[32]

As noted earlier, decisions and decision-making activities permeate almost every human activity. When this human activity is problem-solving, decisions are geared to the identification of a problem, determination of the goal or outcome to be achieved, the prescription of the strategies or methods to be utilized to resolve the problem and to achieve the expected goal, and determination of the outcome.

A goal contains a test or prescription to determine when the predetermined state of affairs has been achieved, in which case the goal is satisfied. A goal is capable of controlling behavior under appropriate conditions—valid and rational attempts to attain the goal. The control takes the form of evolving patterns of behavior that have a rational relation to the goal and to the methods for attaining the goal.[33]

The theory of human problem-solving developed by Newell and Simon is helpful in determining the scope and substance or components of the human problem-solving framework. It explains the *act* of problem-solving and provides a framework that draws on decision, perception, and communication theories and within which these theories flourish.

Dimensions in the variation of the system of the person involved in problem-solving consist of individual differences, man's place on the phylogenetic and time scales, and behavioral acts that include learning, development, and performance. A person is considered to be an information processing system when he is solving problems. As an information processing system, the person behaves through a period of time, with each new act characterized as a function of the immediately preceding state of the person and his environment.[34] When a person is placed in a problem-solving situation and is motivated toward this goal, the behavior is termed adaptive or rational. This behavior is considered to be appropriate to the goal in light of the problem environment and is the behavior demanded by the situation.[35] This includes a person's actual behaviors and the set of possible behaviors from which these are drawn (not only his overt behaviors but also behaviors he thinks of at the time that do not correspond to possible overt behaviors). The space in which his problem-solving activities occur is called the *problem space*. This is not a real space per se, one that can be described as an objective fact for a person. The mere attempt to describe the problem space results in the construction of the *task environment*, the person's representation of the problem.[36]

According to Newell and Simon, when a person is presented with a problem,

> he must encode these problem components—defining goals, rules, and other aspects of the situation—in some kind of space that represents the initial situation to him, the desired goal situation, various intermediate states, imagined or experienced, as well as any concepts he uses to describe these situations to himself.[37]

They propose that the problem space and problem formulation impose organization on the problem-solving process.

A problem can be defined as the situation occurring when a person wants something and does not immediately know what series of actions he can perform to attain it, according to Newell and Simon.

> The desired object may be very tangible (an apple to eat) or abstract (an elegant proof for a theorem). It may be specific . . . or quite general . . . It may be a physical object (an apple) or a set of symbols (the proof of a theorem). The actions involved in obtaining desired objects include physical actions (walking, reaching, writing), perceptual activities (looking, listening), and purely mental activities (judging the similarity of two symbols, remembering a scene, and so on).[38]

Human problem-solving is to be understood by means of describing the task environment in which it takes place, the space the problem solver uses to represent the environment, the task itself, the knowledge about it that is gradually accumulated, and the program the problem solver assembles for approaching the task.[39] The problem solver's program extracts some of the structural information that is embedded in the task environment in order to find solutions by means of a highly selective search through the problem space. The problem space (where problem-solving takes place) contains not only the actual solution but also possible solutions that the problem solver might consider.[40]

The problem space consists of (1) a set of elements that represent a state of knowledge about the task, (2) a set of strategies that produce new states of knowledge from an existing state of knowledge, (3) an initial state of knowledge that is the knowledge about the task that the problem solver has at the start of problem-solving, (4) a problem posed by specifying a set of final desired states to be reached, and (5) the total knowledge available to the problem solver when he is in a given knowledge state. This knowledge state includes (from the most stable information to the most transient) reference information that is constant throughout the course of problem-solving, access information to other knowledge states that have been reached previously and held in long-term memory, path (prior) information about how a given knowledge state was arrived at and what other actions were taken in this state if it has already been visited on prior occasions, access information to the additional symbol structures held in the long-term memory or the extended knowledge state, the knowledge state itself (the dynamic information about the task), and temporary dynamic information created and used exclusively within a single knowledge state.[41]

The problem space may be constructed gradually as the need for the component pieces arises. The assumption that the problem solver is in a fully developed problem space with all of its associated data may be only an estimation of reality.[42]

Regarding the content of the problem solver's knowledge, behavior is not simply a function of a few collective features of this content—how much content there is or how it is expressed. Newell and Simon state,

> Behavior is a function of the specific detail of content of the actual facts of the particular task in hand. And this content governs not just a partial aspect of the behavior of the IPS (information processing system), but all aspects. The behavior of an IPS cannot be understood from syntax alone, abstracted from the vocabulary and semantics of what is being said and done. Methods and programs themselves are content.[43]

It is required that a person as an information processing system must be capable of developing and learning. He is expected to make four principle types of decisions:

1. At a knowledge state (a node in the problem space), to select an operator (strategy) to be applied.
2. At a new knowledge state, to determine whether problem solving shall continue from this state or not.
3. At a knowledge state, to determine whether the knowledge state shall be remembered, so that return can be made to it at some later time.

4. At a decision to abandon a knowledge state, instead of continuing to search for it, to select another knowledge state as a backup state.[44]

Associated with the question of what mechanisms are used to determine actual problem spaces and programs is the question concerning the effect of individual differences. Large individual differences exist that must be reflected in some way in the actual space and program adopted by an individual problem solver for a given occasion. The problem space and specific set of methods used with it need not remain constant through an entire problem-solving attempt.[45]

The task environment (the problem solver's representation of the problem) refers to an environment plus a goal, problem or task—the one for which the motivation of the problem solver is assumed. "It is the task that defines a point of view about an environment, and that, in fact, allows an environment to be delimited." [46] Regarding the task environment, clear distinctions among the environment itself, the internal representation of the task environment used by the problem solver (the problem space), and the objective description of that environment must be made. Problem spaces are defined in relation to task goals, and the representations are restricted to aspects of the total environment that are task relevant.[47] The only aspects of the task environment that are relevant to solving a problem in a particular problem space are those reflected in the structure of that space (the behavior of the problem solver—the nurse, the client—can be described as taking place in the problem space) and the effectiveness of a problem-solving scheme depends completely on its reflecting aspects of the structure of the task environment.[48]

Problem-solving can be effective only if significant information about the objective environment is encoded in the problem space, where it can be used by the problem solver. There can be no guarantee that all the relevant information in the task environment is reflected in the problem space, hence the need to make adaptations as new relevant information becomes available to the problem solver. The task environment remains the overwhelming determinant of the problem space.[49] Newell and Simon state,

> While no precise answer to how a particular problem space used by a problem solver is determined, information about the general intelligence of the problem solver plus his knowledge in relevant domains is often sufficient to predict what problem space he will use. Thus, the task environment remains the overwhelming determinant of the problem space.[50]

To summarize, then, the problem space and the problem formation impose an overall organization on the problem-solving process utilized by the problem solver. The process is initiated with the translation of input by the problem solver. This produces for the problem solver an internal representation of the external environment, and, at the same time, a selection of a problem space. The problem solver then proceeds within the framework of the internal representation thus produced—a representation that may render problem solutions obvious, obscure, or perhaps unattainable. For example, the problem solver may simply recognize the answer to the problem. The answer recognized was already in the memory of the problem solver or was simply evoked by the act of understanding the question. Recognition processes are important for solving problems not only because they can be used in the solution of difficult problems, but also because problem-solving often proceeds by reduction. In other words, a difficult problem is reduced to something the problem solver already knows. The result is immediate when a problem is solved by recognition.[51]

This theory focuses on the collection of information processes that combine a series of means to an end, or at least an attempt to attain an end.

> The means that are usable by a problem solving system are dictated by the nature of the internal representation, for specifying a problem space determines the various ways in which the initial situation can be changed to reach the goal situation. Ends arise out of the formulation of goals or subgoals . . . A method can be understood only in reference to its goal . . . A method, then is tied closely to its associated problem formulation. The method resides in the problem solver prior to its evocation to deal with any individual task. Thus, the method can be fashioned without specific knowledge of the particular problem situations it will be called upon to handle. Consequently, mechanisms must exist in the problem solver for bringing the problem solving method into effective correspondence with each individual problem situation, so that the method can actually discover something about the situation and act upon it.[52]

As the problem is represented internally, the system responds by relating a particular problem-solving method or strategy. In addition to the recognition method mentioned previously there are a variety of methods that could serve as the means to achieve the end. A trial and error, or generate and test, method may be used in which potential solutions are tested until one resolves the problem. Another method involves the generation of possible solutions to guide the search based on information garnered sequentially. This method or strategy bears some rational relation to attaining a problem solution, as formulated and seen in terms of the internal representation. The selected strategies are applied (which eventually control the internal and external behavior of the problem solver). Such is the case when a nursing diagnosis is made and the prescribed strategies are designed to offset the client problem and then implemented, thus bringing about a change in client behavior in a preferred direction toward optimal wellness.

The symbol structure belonging to the method becomes a particularized problem formulation. "It communicates to the method what information is known about the specific problem situation and thus provides the *givens* that the method requires in order to execute its processes. Thus, a method is inextricably interwoven with its problem formulation." [53]

At any moment during which the outcome of either the processes incorporated in the method or strategy itself or of the general processes that monitor its application and achievement of the goal, the execution of the method or strategy may be halted. When a method or strategy is terminated, the problem solver has three options: (1) another method may be attempted, (2) the problem may be reformulated, or (3) the attempt to solve the problem may be abandoned.[54]

During its operation, a method or strategy may produce new problems (subgoals) and the problem solver may elect to attempt to solve one of these. The problem solver also has the option of setting aside a new subgoal, continuing instead with another branch of original method or strategy. There is a continuous influx of new information from the external environment that may offer new solution possibilities or demands that cause the problem solver to interrupt current activities to try different ones. At a more detailed perceptual level—scanning of task environment or interval representation—the problem solver may see many things simultaneously, but takes action on only one at a time.[55] The problem solver's behavior will be circular in character, consisting of repeated loops around a circuit—select a goal—select a method or strategy—evaluate results—select a goal. Note the similarity to the nursing process.

Difficulties in problem-solving can be measured in a variety of ways, i.e., whether or not a solution is attained, the time required to find a solution, and the quality of the solution, to mention a few. Problem difficulty will be determined by the interaction between the task environment and the method or strategy of the information processing system of the problem solver. The size of the problem space provides one key to the estimation of problem difficulty. The problem space defines the set of possibilities for the solution as seen by the problem solver. Time measured from problem designation to solution will be roughly proportional to the total size of the problem space. The initial space in which the problem solver encodes the problem provides a measure of the size of a problem world. As each piece of relevant information is applied (either information contained in the problem specification or already stored in the problem solver's memory), the problem solver diminishes the size of the problem space by restricting himself to a more relevant subspace. The problem solver may not know how to use information to reduce the space. After as much reduction as possible is achieved there may be a subspace that cannot be reduced further because the problem solver has no more relevant information. At this point, a method must be adopted that requires the examination of all the elements of the remaining subspace. Two problem solvers at about the same level of intelligence and ability will detect and use approximately the same information in going from the space where they initially formulate the problem to the space where they actually apply their problem-solving methods. The demands of the situation will be essentially the same for both. However, problem solvers who have widely different levels of intelligence, knowledge, and ability may achieve different reductions in the subspace and thereby face different problem demands.[56]

Einstein and Infeld state in *The Evolution of Physics* that the formulation of a problem is often far more essential than its solution, which may be merely a matter of mathematical or experimental skills. They believe that to raise new questions, new possibilities, and to regard old problems from a new angle requires creative imagination and marks a real advance in science.[57]

When a group of individuals, such as a nursing team, must jointly choose a strategy or course of action related to decision making and problem-solving, it is understood that although it is a cohesive group, there are different preferences for outcomes that not only jointly affect, but may also differ in the personal probability assessments for different possible events. The differences in the knowledge, understanding, and skills of the group or team members will exert an impact.

In a given situation (including a nursing situation) individuals may agree both on the utility values of the consequences and on the conditional probability assessments for different outcomes for a given underlying condition. Group members may disagree on their assessments of probabilities for the underlying states, e.g., they may disagree on the client's nursing diagnosis. They can either "(1) compromise on a prior distribution over these states before they take their sample and then use the sample results to update their group prior distribution or (2) each individual can use the sample results to get his very own posterior probability distribution and then all the individuals can compromise the differences . . ."[58] The democratic process, the utilization of a panel of experts, additional knowledge, and specialized help are some of the means that could be utilized to resolve differences and bring about an effective compromise.

Any particular strategy or method to be used may be described in terms of a set of scaled values, such as comfort, convenience, value to the client or to the nurse, logic, economy, and convenience to both client and nurse. Decision analysis usually begins with a listing of all the possible strategies for experimentation and action, then an evaluation of each strategy, which is conditional on the state of the world, and finally an averaging of these conditional evaluations by weighing the states according to their judgmental probabilities. Common sense and simple mathematical analysis, or both, may make it possible to find a reasonably small set of strategies that is guaranteed to contain the best, or optimal, strategy or strategies sought by the problem solver. Some of the strategies or alternatives could be eliminated after careful and systematic reflection. The decision makers and problem solvers reflect on the remaining alternatives, refining measurements, adding more possibilities, and extending the breadth and depth of the decision analysis. Eventually more strategies can safely be eliminated while continuing the process of embellishment, refinement and extension, and maximizing the utility values and probability until the optimal strategy or strategies are determined for implementation.[59]

When problem-solving continues over an extended period of time, it is practical and productive to combine an extensive form of decision analysis with a modified analysis. This is particularly evident when considering problems in which the effects of action taken in the present will linger over a long period of time (10–20 years, as, for example, client problems resulting from chronic illness). Decision analysis continues for the present and an immediate future of 1–2 or 2–3 or 3–5 years. Raiffa believes it is a challenge to shorten the time comprising a distant future and convert it into an immediate future for decision-making and problem-solving purposes.[60]

Thus, one goal in the deliberative use of the nursing process is to solve a problem. The nursing process can be used to design a course of action aimed at changing an existing situation into a preferred one. Solving a problem means representing it in a manner such that its solution becomes transparent.[61] The more difficult and novel the problem is, the more likely trial and error will be required to find a solution. Trial and error, or generate and test, methods are highly selective and represent progress toward a goal. Indications of progress spur further search in the same direction whereas a lack of progress is a signal to look elsewhere for the solution. This is another way of demonstrating the cyclic nature of the nursing process with its built-in evaluation component, determining progress toward a goal. If the goal is not reached, then the course of action must be modified and reassessed. Problem-solving requires selective trial and error. A decision is made as to which path to try first and what data are promising.[62] Simon states that when we examine sources from which the problem-solving system derives its selectivity, that selectivity can always be equated with some kind of information feedback from the environment. There are basically two kinds of selectivity: (a) various paths are tried and consequences noted; this information is used as a guide to further search, and (b) previous experience. When a problem to be solved is comparable to one resolved previously, similar paths may again be tried. Given a desired and an existing state, the task of an adaptive organism is to find the difference between these two states and the correlating process that would erase the difference. The task is to discover a sequence of processes that would produce the desired goal from the initial state. The activity of human problem-solving is a form of means-to-an-end analysis aimed at discovering a process description of the path that leads to a desired goal.[63] The nursing process is such a process. The primacy of goal-attainment, as a function of a system, gives priority to processes involved most directly with the success or failure of goal-oriented endeavors.

Inherent in problem-solving activity are choices, decisions about choices, and decisions about decisions.

When a problem is recognized, defined, and solved, the perception as well as the value system of the decision maker should be considered. Values give significance and meaning to the problem and determine the degree and nature of the action to be taken.[64] The ability to perceive problems is also related to knowledge of that area in which the problem is located. The problem-solving process includes that by which a person implements or makes a decision work. It is recognized as a continuing dynamic process rather than as an occasional event. All judgments that affect a course of action are decisions. The value of a decision stems from the degree to which goals are achieved.

The crucial stage in the problem-solving process is the evaluation of proposed solutions to the problem, because it is at this point that the value system and aspirations of the decision maker have an impact on the process. The selection of a solution is only part of the process that resulted after several solutions or decisions were formulated, the consequences weighed or probabilities assigned to each, and the solution most likely to be successful selected. The evaluation stems from the purpose for which the solution was proposed or the reason why the decision was made. During the implementation phase of the decision process, numerous minor decisions may have to be made to modify the solution, as dictated by continuous feedback as the solution becomes operational.[65]

To enhance the caliber of the decisions made, policies may be established that set limitations on the manner and content of decision making. These limitations include the purpose of the system or subsystem, the criterion of rationality of action of members or parts of a system, relevant information, lines of communication, role designations, and time limits.[66] Decision making and problem solving are sequential processes. Each step in these processes is based on previous ones. As new information is introduced, the direction of the sequence will change. A decision has an impact on action, in that a course of action may be altered, reversed, discontinued, or continued.[67]

Theoretical formulations from game theory support decision and problem-solving theories and add a dimension to the understanding of the problem-solving process. The theory of games is based on a sequence of moves or strategies, made by different players, according to a prescribed order, which may depend on the choices made and their outcomes. Either a strategy or the probability of a number of strategies exists for each player. The advantage of communication and cooperation in some games in which players may achieve a pay-off is obvious. The strategies chosen, then, are those most likely to be of maximum benefit to the players. If the nurse and the client are viewed as players in a game geared to meet the goals of each, communication and cooperation between nurse and client may facilitate the selection of those strategies or means by which both can achieve their goals or pay-off.[68]

A decision or choice is based on the examination of strategies and the range of possible outcomes. The decision maker or problem solver is a complex, living, behaving, goal-seeking system. The living, behaving, adaptive systems of nurse and client are open, both internally and externally, and are negentropic. The interchanges and interactions between systems may cause changes in the nature of each system or subsystem. These changes may have significant implications for the whole system.[69] Internal and external exchanges are transferred by the flow of information (via chemical, cortical, social, or cultural encoding and decoding). Feedback-control facilitates self-regulation and self-direction. Thus the system may change its structure to insure its survival or viability.

Perception Theory

In a thriving, living, behaving system in which matter, energy, and information are exchanged within the system as well as with its environment, perception plays an important role. Theories shed light on the origin of the process of perception and provide a rationale for perceptive awareness of the interaction between internal and external environments of the living behaving system or person. The decisions a person makes and his awareness of the choices available to him in a given situation are influenced by his perception of himself as he creates an environment for himself through which he achieves satisfaction and fulfills certain goals. Each person deals with situations according to his own unique system of behavior. Consequently, different persons may view a given situation differently and each person will assume that which he perceives is real.

In considering perception, its relationship to the nervous system and the extent to which some aspects of perception do not depend on learning and experience are significant. Day states that perception can be studied in terms of three sets of variables: those in the physical environment, physiologic processes and interactions, and behavioral events. Aspects of perception that serve to mediate overt behavioral responses are the combined function of neural storage, peripheral activity, and central neural events. Central neural storage is a term used to designate the repository of an individual's past as well as current stimulation, with attendant responses resulting in neural events and changes. The overt response of an individual gives rise to kinesthetic, muscular, and mechanical stimulation. The total stimulus complex constitutes a feedback system from response to stimulus input.[70]

Contact between man and his environment is accomplished by energy sensitive receptors specifically responsive to certain forms of energy. The characteristics of the stimulation must be transformed into a code for transmission to higher levels of the central nervous system before contact can be established and appropriate adaptive responses initiated. This reception, followed by transformation and energy coding, is the first stage of the perceptual process.[71]

Three classes of receptor cells have been proposed: exteroceptors, interoceptors, and proprioceptors. Exteroceptors are those sensory organ cells that receive energy from the external environment. Interoceptors are cells that respond to changes in pressure, temperature, and pain, including changes in bodily organs and systems within the organism. Proprioceptors are sensitive to energy changes caused by activities involving movement and posture. These three classes of receptor cells selectively pick up stimuli consisting of the total energy changes that occur in the environment, within the organism itself, or that are induced by the activities of the organism.[72] Only restricted ranges of environmental energy are necessary to activate the receptors. Also, energy must vary over either time or space; if the stimulus does not change, receptors adapt and become insensitive to it. (Recall the reactions of clients to sensory deprivation and overload during care in highly technical areas of health care facilities.) The sensory system converts the energy of the stimulus and encodes its various properties.[73]

A framework to define perception as developed by Day follows. Perception is considered in terms of variables in the physical environment, physiologic processes and interactions, and behavioral events. Stimulus variables are those that occurred in the person's past as well as current stimulation. Past stimulation, with its attendant responses, results in neural events and changes that can be termed *central neural storage*. A currently acting stimulus induces processes in both the peripheral nervous system (receptors and their structures), called *peripheral neural activity*, and in the central regions (including the cerebral cortex), called *central neural activity*. Central neural storage, peripheral neural activity, and central neural events can be thought of as combining to produce the phenomenal events of perception. These events serve to mediate the overt behavioral response, which gives rise to kinesthetic and muscular stimulation. Mechanical stimulation from the individual's activity is included as part of the total stimulus complex. This constitutes a feedback system from the response to stimulus input.[74] Numerous theories have contributed to an understanding of these perceptual components or events.

Perception may be determined in large part by the learned meanings given to stimuli. Meanings may be inherent in a certain property of stimulation or they may be given by labeling, or by an expectancy induced in the observer. Meanings that are learned affect perception the most when the conditions under which stimulation occurs are ambiguous.[75] Simple percepts lead to more complex perceptual processes associated with the identification of objects, which, in turn, lead to organized perception formed by learning, manipulating, and memorizing previous events.[76]

A perceptive person builds up strong probabilities concerning many expected features of the environment. These greatly affect the particular environmental cues he selects at any one moment for perception and judgment. By checking the accuracy of his percepts by means of his actions (feedback), he is able to select those cues most likely to give correct or truthful information about the nature of objects and environment. Spatial relationships, locations, colors, distance, movement, would serve as examples.[77] Usually an abundance of information is available and contributes to minimizing error. The process of perception is integrated with processes of identification, classification, and coding. These processes depend on learning, memory, attention, reasoning, and language. Simple perceptual processes provide data for the operation of more complex processes.[78] Accuracy may be lost when the data are systematized and identified because certain features are ignored, distorted, or over- or under-emphasized. The person must learn to employ the data obtained by perception in such a way that it effectively improves his ability to discriminate. These data may be organized and integrated into complex perceptual systems. The ability to perceive form, position, and the movement of objects in relation to the position and movement of the body is enormously important in understanding adjustments to normal surroundings.[79] To maintain normal perception and cognition, one must be able to perceive change and variation as they occur. The results of research point to profound changes that may result from exposure to homogeneous and unvarying stimulation over a long period of time. The effects of sensory deprivation on the client are apparent to the nurse. This holds true, in a dramatic way, for the client who is unconscious or isolated for some reason. Perception tends to become increasingly less accurate during long periods of observing or responding to a monotonous, repeated stimulation. Many have experienced this impact after they have driven for long, uninterrupted periods on high-speed roadways. There is a physiologic basis for the decrease in alertness and attention due to unvarying stimulation. The discovery of the reticular formation of the brain stem and thalamus, with its variable function, under different types of stimulation, and the control it exercises on cortical functions related to perception, supports the probability that direct attention to various aspects of the environment is related to reticular formation function. This, in turn, may be affected by motivational processes.[80]

Perhaps other cognitive functions may be involved in these complex perceptual processes. It has been shown that information is rarely derived simply from instantaneous perceptions that fade immediately from memory. Impressions are prolonged, at least for a short time, in the primary memory image. This provides continuity in our perceptions of the environment and enhances the use of remembered past experiences as well as the application of reasoning and judgment in evaluating events before reacting or deciding how to act or react. Coding single stimuli and classifying isolated events into perceptual designs provides the basis for understanding the nature of the environment. Life experiences are seldom a function of isolated events but are determined by the continuity of knowledge and experience associated with such perceptions. The inferences a person makes about the nature of objects and events involves knowledge and experiences.[81]

In many life situations, immediate perception may be incorporated in and supplemented by deliberation, judgment, and decision. Individual differences are apparent in many types of perception. People may perceive and react effectively to stimulation without being clearly aware of their total operative percepts. The various reactions demonstrated by different individuals in response to the same situation—witnesses to an accident—supports this statement. Inferences and judgments related to percepts of these witnesses would be as varied as the number of individuals. Motivation and emotion have an effect on arousing, directing, facilitating, or inhibiting the perception of relevant situations and events. But differences in knowledge and acquired skill, of intelligence and ability, are of greater importance than motivational influences in directing attention and promoting efficient discrimination. Accurate perception of the environment is essential to preserve life. Although perception may be partially selective, to perform its essential functions efficiently, the selection cannot vary with individual disposition more than to a minor extent.[82]

Vernon also points out that prolonged deprivation of sensory stimulation, and, perhaps even more, of perceptual stimulation, may have far-reaching effects on the normal functioning of cognitive processes. These effects are more severe in some persons than in others. She further states that not only is perception likely to be most rapid and accurate in relevant situations, but expectations are established in such a manner that attention is quickly aroused and directed effectively toward these situations as soon as they occur. While there is a tendency to respond to novel and unexpected events, more deliberate perception and inference may be necessary to gain a full understanding of the situation before action takes place. A fundamental tendency is the ability to respond to a constantly varying environment. Movement is considered a frequent environmental variation. It is supposed that there is an innate tendency to perceive the movements of people. It is possible that learning through experiences may influence the inception of these perceptions—as in the perception of smiling faces. These perceptions can be enormously refined and improved through learning.[83]

Vernon concludes that perception begins with the responses of cell units in the sensory mechanism to stimuli. These responses are then integrated into patterns and configurations that are fundamentally significant in perception. She hypothesizes that the infant possesses an innate tendency to perceive form as well as the natural environment in terms of objects and that this tendency begins to operate as his experiences with objects develop. The infant has a natural tendency to perceive a spatial continuum within which objects are spatially related to himself and to each other. It is supposed that from infancy upwards, the child builds up complex integrations (also called schemata) by means of which what is perceived at any moment is related to memories and knowledge, particularly those obtained through the active experience of manipulating objects and moving through the environment.[84] The process of reasoning and of conceptual classification comes to bear on these integrations.

Perception of objects, particularly in the complex environmental settings with which we are normally concerned, develops comparatively slowly. This development depends on the capacity to sort out essential aspects from a multitude of irrelevant detail. The nature and identity of new and unfamiliar objects are explored and discovered by the child himself by applying not only his habitual activities but also variations of these to find out what can be done with the objects. Carefully, he watches to see what happens to an object when he lets it fall to the floor. He forms a notion of what action to perform and what its outcome may be. Integration or schemata of perception are involved, covering categories of objects (appearance, behavior, use) associated together as they relate to each other in complex organizations. Immediate perception is integrated with respect to conceptual reasoning.[85] The capacity to extract such general qualities as size, number, volume, weight, height, and to judge these, irrespective of the objects and settings in which they occur, requires reasoning. This is an essential component of judgment and involves the realization that these attributes may remain constant in spite of changes in appearance or setting. Vernon gives a useful example of this idea when she notes that the volume of water remains constant when it is poured from a wide container into a narrow one, even though the level of water in the latter is higher. A child may observe the obvious height of the water level. His judgment of the volume of water in the container is overweighted by his perception of the water level, and he may note that the volume of water is different. There are other situations in which immediate perception is uncorrected by reasoning.[86]

Vernon continues her discussion of perception through experiences by stating that the ability to modify immediate perception through reasoning is generally supposed to develop as a person matures, although at the stage at which it begins to develop, experience and learning may affect it considerably. While the capacity to identify and recognize is determined by maturation to a considerable extent, experience is known to play an important role, providing information about the nature and characteristics of objects.[87] The identification of these objects—general qualities and types—is based on information.

The following suppositions relate to perception through experience:

1. Generalization of learning from one situation to another could occur in so far as situations or events become organized within the same schemata in a manner such that present percepts are filled out and extended by memories of relevant past experiences and appropriate responses are made available.
2. The utilization of class categories is a significant feature of improved identification from the second year of life. Children and adults learn to distinguish the invariant qualities of a class of events or objects (on which identification is based) from chance variations resulting from changes in the background situation.
3. Verbal discrimination plays a significant role in the process

> of naming, labeling, and coding. Verbal information furthers the control of immediate perception by reasoning processes.[88]

It does not necessarily follow, even if one perceives with a reasonable degree of accuracy or truthfulness, that shapes and contours are exact replicas of the stimulus pattern falling on the eye. The forms of which persons are actually aware may be reconstructions from sensory data. There are many aspects of complex situations provided by the natural environment of which persons are not accurately aware. The stimulus pattern gives rise to cues from which the appearance of objects and their spatial setting can be inferred. Perceptions of form in everyday life may not involve accurate discrimination of minute detail, although the capacity to do this is available. This capacity may be utilized in selected scientific activities or in precision measurements. Generally there is an overabundance of sensory information, much of which is corroborative. The observer must select what is relevant to his identification of the objects and events he visualizes and initiate appropriate reaction. The perceiver utilizes schematized knowledge as to the type of situation and the relevant response pattern. There may be occasions in which information is restricted or conflicting. It may be so abundant that one must sift for relevancy and discard that which is irrelevant. In situations such as this, the perceiver makes inferences about the real nature of the situation or about the objects presented to him.[89] The nurse experiences this when she must gather data on an unconscious person and no one is available to give information about his predicament. Other examples are data available about an infant if there is no adult with him to interpret, or if a person—either the nurse or the client—speaks a foreign language, a highly technical language, or if the language is distorted. By making inferences the observer goes beyond immediate sensory data and extracts information that gives the truest impression of the nature of the situation in which immediately perceptible aspects of the stimulus occur. Inference may override erroneous impressions given by visual illustrations.[90] There are conditions, however, in which inferences related to the identity of objects and events are erroneous; for example, those seen in dim light, from great distances, or for short periods of time. In terms of the perception of words, understanding their meaning seems to be more important than their frequency.[91]

The relationship between attention and perception has been studied by some investigators who have demonstrated that there may be a process of attending that operates independently of perceptual processes. Previously, it was thought that if a person attended a stimulus, he automatically perceived it. Physiologic and psychologic investigations have identified a special center in the brain that is concerned with attention. A decline in attention and in interference with normal perception has been noted in persons partially or completely deprived of variable sensory stimulation.[92]

While observers are prone to make inferences from fragments of information and these inferences are influenced by what the observer expects to perceive, focusing attention on particular events or aspects of the stimulus, and the expectation that certain types of stimulation may occur, may identify stimuli which, under other circumstances, would be ignored completely.[93]

The implications for the nurse are many. Continual striving to increase the observational field, as well as to increase her knowledge about human behavior and the human situation, could enhance her ability to collect data and increase the accuracy of her inferences concerning the client. Thus, she can make educated estimates about gaps in data and pursue specific information to fill them. The process used to select data, reactions to data or stimuli, and her focus on particular events related to the availability or absence of data is a decision process.

While the foregoing discussion has centered more on perception as it relates to form, objects, languages, space, and movement, an important perceptual schema that differs considerably is the perception of people, their emotions, and their actions. Vernon believes that from the earliest years people perceived other people, their faces, and their behavior in a manner unique to these types of percepts. A special schemata has evolved within which these percepts are integrated. The unique aspect of these percepts is that the perceivers are mainly aware of the intentions, emotions, and personality characteristics of persons; only to a minor extent are they aware of the details of the physical characteristics (appearance and behavior) of these people. Stimulus patterns involved in the perception of persons are more complex and extensive than those on which the perception of objects is based. From early infancy, previous knowledge and expectations concerning the actions and motives of people are highly significant, and from their perceptions of physical properties, children learn to make inferences about significant characteristics of people and their behavior.[94] As they develop their perception of persons, infants and children look predominantly into the eyes and upper part of a person's face. Relative to the perception of emotion, facial expressions related to somewhat temporary emotions are differentiated from perceptions of more lasting characteristics by which familiar people are identified and impressions of their personality characteristics are based. Emotions frequently felt and expressed may give rise to permanent facial characteristics, such as wrinkles around the eyes and in the forehead.[95]

In reference to the accuracy with which emotional expressions are perceived, studies indicate that emotions judged from facial expressions are easier to differentiate if they correspond to the extremes of pleasant/unpleasant or attention/rejection. This does not mean that this is the extent to which perceptions of emotional expressions are accurate in everyday situations. Facial expression is a dynamic and constantly changing characteristic. It is accompanied by action, expressive gestures, and changes in vocal intonation. Studies have shown that infants understand the emotions of others, i.e., fear, anger. Of course, this depends on whether the relationship between the emotion that is felt and its outward expression is consistent.[96]

Perceptual data on which assessments of emotions other than one's own are based are extremely complex. It is difficult, if not impossible, to isolate any one facial feature that is consistently associated with a particular emotional expression. Some expressions can be identified readily, such as a smile or a frown. There seems to be little basis for some prevailing associations—a high forehead indicates high intelligence, for example. Again, the implication is obvious, in that far-reaching judgments or inferences, based on little or selected data, may be totally inaccurate. Prejudices and stereotypes have resulted from this tendency to select certain facial characteristics and bodily poses. Some associations between facial and personality characteristics may result in social stereotypes. It is generally considered, for example, that a smiling face with an uncurved mouth indicates a good-tempered person. These stereotyped associations vary in different societies and in different groups within these societies. Often, stereotypes are more likely to be attributed to strangers or foreigners. The more resemblance there is between a stranger and a familiar person the more likely the stereotype will be favorable.[97]

Floyd Allport [98] contributed some insights to the understanding of the nature of perception when he analyzed it from a systems viewpoint. He compares organisms and machines (cybernetics) and notes that each has a common feature—input and output. For the organism, input is the stimulus (energy, food, water), whereas output is the work done by the effector or mechanism. The system's internal operation is akin to metabolism—that point of operation connecting input and output. Psychologically speaking, input would refer to the energy derived from stimulated receptors whereas output is the coordination of the action of effectors called *behaviors.* Both machines and organisms use working energy, power, and raw materials as input and convert this to service and finished product as outputs. There are special energetic units that usually operate through some subsystem referred to as *information.* This information can be compared to the stimulations received by the organism through its receptors, since it affects the action of the machine or organism in a controlled manner. Random stimuli or energetic events that do not become effective toward output bombard the organism, and are referred to as *noise.* Information that affects output is considered negative entropy or organization; random disturbances of noise are entropy. The designer of a machine strives to keep noise to a minimum while the organism (particularly the human organism) strives to reduce the proportion of random, uncoordinated, or disorganized behavior through perception, reasoning, or learning.[99]

Human beings communicate with and control one another, within the organization of society, by spoken word, and by using mechanical transmitting devices, such as the telephone or telegraph. Information can be communicated to a machine to fulfill a task. The communicator of information to parts or subsystems of a mechanical system enables the parts to be synchronized to the demands of the task—rate of output is controlled by the system to contribute to purposeful goals. The feedback mechanism enhances the interdependence of parts of the system, keeping it in a steady state as the flow from input goes through it. Its function is to regulate and control the operation of the entire system. The amount of information fed back to the main part of the system is always equal to the extent to which there remains a gap between the actual and desired condition. It corrects many fluctuations in the operation of a complicated mechanism, with a minimal amount of inefficiency or loss. The feedback principle is prevalent in natural, socially evolved, and deliberately constructed systems.[100]

The living organism has an input and an output. It has receptors into which information is fed. There are effectors in the organism—muscles, glands, etc., as well as an arrangement for integrating, storing, and transferring information between input and output. Storage and recollection are located in the physiologic mechanism through which information is retained, recognized, and recalled. Messages are not only transmitted from the outside but also from within the system through established pathways. These messages are delivered by the kinesthetic receptors and proprioceptors of the organism. The nervous system, like the computer, operates on relatively small amounts of energy in which the structural character of the operations is circular rather than linear.[101] But, the operator designates the purpose and is the basis for the feedback subsystem. The purpose is not in any part of the system, but is the end for which the system was designed.

If living behaving systems are viewed as aggregates of designated ongoing events, they will be found to have a selflimited, self-enclosed, and circular character. These same forms of events apply to systems at a higher level—to all collective or societal aggregates in which organisms operate, including economic, political, and other systems in which men or machines play a part. Circular operating structures may be conceived as interrelated by the same set of principles that enter into their individual construction and operation.[102] Thus, systems theory, particularly theories related to machine and communication systems, shed some light on the study of the nature and process of perception. These theories have enhanced the knowledge of how the brain and nervous system operate.

To understand meaning in perception, one must approach it through the perceived character of objects and situations that have meaning for us. There are other phases of meaning, but that which gives us the unique characteristics of objects and situations is the one most central to the entire perceptual process. Meaning has a wider scope than the perceived character of objects. It enters into processes in addition to that of perception. Meaning is the very appropriateness with which perceiving, remembering, and acting are explained. When we perceive, remember, think, or will, we assign meaning.[103] Thus, perception plays a crucial role in life in general, for it is the sole means by which we can gather information about the world around us. It is also the only means by which nurse and client gather data about each other. In turn, these data are assigned designated values and then used to fulfill the purposes of nursing.

Human Need Theory

After presentation of the theoretical formulations within which the nursing process exists, it follows that the *theoretical substance* of the nursing process must be defined. This substance is drawn from human need and motivation theories. It is believed that the *preser-*

vation of, the fostering of, the maintenance of, and the facilitation of the integrity of all of the human needs of the person(s) is the territory of nursing.

The works of Maslow and Montagu provide the theoretical substance for the understanding of human needs and the motivation inherent in meeting these needs.[104, 105] The earlier works of such persons as Bronislaw Malinowski, Laurence Kubie, G. L. Freeman, and Ralph Clinton are acknowledged for their contributions to the development of human need theory.[106, 107, 108, 109]

Proponents of human need theory view the person as an integrated, organized whole who is motivated toward meeting his basic human needs. A human need is viewed as an internal tension that results from an alteration in some state of the system. This tension expresses itself in goal-directed behavior of the person that continues until goal satisfaction (freedom from tension) is achieved.[110] A basic or vital human need is one that must be satisfied if the person or the group is to survive.[111] The nurse's role encompasses completely basic or vital human needs and their satisfaction for herself and the client, although the fulfillment of one or a selection of human needs poses problems for the client due to biologic, intellectual, emotional, social, spiritual, economic, environmental, pathophysiologic, and psychopathologic affronts.

Preconditions to assure health and humanness include physical, chemical, biologic, psychologic, interpersonal, and cultural conditions that either do or do not supply the person with the basic necessities and rights that allow him to develop his strength and humanity to the degree that facilitates his assumption of responsibility for his own fate. Maslow believes that the actualization of a person's full and real potential is further conditioned by the presence of parents and other persons who satisfy basic human needs, ecologic and cultural factors fostering health, and by the situation in the world at large.[112] Health with all of its values, truth, goodness, and beauty is viewed as an attainable, real state.

A person is motivated by human needs for air, food, water, sleep, movement or activity, for safety and escape from danger, protection and care, freedom from pain, for gregariousness and affection, interdependence, love relationships, for respect, standing in relation to others and within his group, status with the consequent self-respect, and by the need for self-fulfillment and realization of the full potential of the individual (self-actualization). Self-actualization is confined to the adult. In addition, a person has cognitive needs for knowledge, curiosity, and understanding (philosophic, theologic, and ethical and value system). A person has aesthetic needs—beauty, symmetry, simplicity, completion, order, as well as the need to express, act out, and for motor accomplishment related to these aesthetic needs.[113, 114]

Maslow emphasizes the holism of the person when he states that most drives cannot be isolated or localized somatically, or considered as if they were the only things happening. "The typical drive or need or desire is not and probably never will be related to a specific, isolated, localized somatic base. The typical desire is much more obviously a need of the whole person." [115] From anthropologic evidence, he concludes that *fundamental or ultimate desires of all human beings do not differ as much as do their conscious everyday desires.*[116]

It is believed that it is normal for an act or conscious wish to have more than one motivation. Maslow believes that fundamental goals or needs, rather than a listing of drives, provide a framework for the construction of motivational life. "Human motivation rarely actualizes itself in behavior except in relation to the situation and to other people." [117] Of course, consideration must be given to the person as an integrated whole in addition to his character structure. A person is considered to be most unified or complete in his integration when he is successfully facing and experiencing a great joy, or a creative moment, or a problem, a threat or an emergency. If the threat is overwhelming, however, or if the person feels weak or helpless, disintegration rather than integration may occur.[118]

A person is motivated to gratify his basic or vital human needs—to seek what is required for need fulfillment. A five-level hierarchical structure is used by Maslow to designate human needs with consideration given (from first to fifth level) to physical needs, safety needs, belonging and love needs, esteem needs, and finally to self-actualization. This contrasts with the two-structure hierarchy specified by Montagu, namely, vital basic human needs and nonvital basic human needs.

Any number of fundamental physical needs may be delineated, with varied degrees of specificity stated. Generally, physical needs relate to air, food, fluids, sleep, rest, sex, exercise and activity, elimination, stimulation, excitement, and maternal response. These needs are relatively independent of each other and have a localized somatic base. These are comparable to the vital human needs delineated by Montagu, which include the need to inhale air, ingest food, take in liquid, rest, be active, sleep, micturate, defecate, escape from danger, and a craving for internal equilibrium. Sex is not viewed as a vital basic need because a person can survive in perfect health without its satisfaction. But it is clearly a need that must be satisfied by some members if the group is to survive.[119, 120]

The physical needs and the consuming behavior involved with their fulfillment serve as channels for other needs as well. These physical needs are viewed as the most influential of all needs in that if a person were lacking in food, safety, love, and esteem, he would most probably hunger for food to a greater extent and more strongly than anything else. This is supported by Montagu in his explanation of basic human needs and their vital sequences. The physiologic tension of oxygen hunger results in the need or urge to take in air, which leads to the act of breathing, resulting in oxygenation of tissues. This restores equilibrium, homeostasis. Or, the physiologic tension of fright results in the urge or need to escape, which leads to the act of escaping from danger and results in relaxation. A person is dominated by physical needs; if all needs are unsatisfied, all other needs may seem nonexistent or be relegated to low priority. If a person is overcome by severe fluid loss and is thirsty or is starving, all human capacity is directed toward restoration of normal fluid balance with effective replacement of affected electrolytes and toward obtaining food. Of these two needs, the need for water may, at times, be a more pressing need than the need for food. The nurse will readily acknowledge these human states from personal or client experiences.[121, 122]

Gratification and deprivation are important concepts in motivation theory. Higher needs emerge when physical or vital basic human needs are reasonably well satisfied. This is the reason for the organization of needs in a hierarchy—beginning first with the powerful physical or vital human needs.

Need fulfillment dominates human activity to the extent that the behavior of the person is organized only in relation to unsatisfied needs. For example, if sleep deprivation occurs and restful sleep ensues, the need becomes relatively unimportant in the dynamics of the person. Maslow points out that it is precisely those persons in whom a certain need has always been met or satisfied who are best equipped to withstand deprivation of that particular need at some future time. Persons who have been deprived in the past will respond differently to current need satisfaction than the person who has never been deprived.[123]

Safety needs emerge when physical needs are gratified. Safety needs include security, stability, dependency, protection, freedom from fear and anxiety, and structure. Montagu's specification of the need to escape from danger may be equated with the safety needs expressed by Maslow—freedom from fear. Safety needs incorporate the need for structure, law, order, limits, and the strength of a protecting person. These basic human needs encompass a person's current outlook of the world and his philosophy of living, including his focus for the future. In times of threat or danger, self-preservation and the need to assure safety and protection become paramount. In fact, practically every other need (including at times the formerly satisfied physical needs) appears to be less important. If a person is held at gunpoint by someone intent on causing fatal injury or if an infant is disturbed, dropped suddenly, hurt, startled, or handled roughly, he will respond to the danger. Little thought in these intense moments will be given to food, sleep, rest, etc. The reaction of infants to threat or danger is spontaneous, total and uninhibited and, therefore, more obvious than in adults who are expected to cover up this response.[124, 125]

Human beings need undisrupted routine and rhythm. They thrive in a predictable, lawful, peaceful and orderly world. They flourish early in life within the encompassing nurturing and protective function of parents and normal family settings. Disruptions within the family relationships due to quarreling, physical assault, separation, abandonment, divorce, or death may be especially devastating. Children, particularly, respond with terror when confronted with new, unfamiliar, strange, and unmanageable stimuli and situations. All of us can recall the response of the child who becomes lost in a department store. The impact of hospitalization on children is well known to nurses. This impact is particularly devastating (perhaps even irreversible) if parents are restricted by health agency policy, in terms of visiting hours, from participation in protecting, caring, and comforting, or separated by structures or partitions, room dividers, or lack of space, so that what is familiar, safe, and known from the child's viewpoint is restricted from view. This situation may be duplicated for aged persons who can no longer manage their affairs and who move to unfamiliar environments. As will be noted later, this situation could contribute to the lack of fulfillment of love and belonging needs as well. Loss of the parental role of protection, new tasks, being confronted with strangers, uncontrollable objects, illness, or death are threats to the need for safety.[126]

Safety needs are expressed when a person seeks a peaceful, smoothly running, stable, good social system that provides a safe environment for its members—one protected from dangerous insects and animals, harmful organisms, odors, chemicals, and related substances, extremes of temperature, humidity level, one free from environmental, technical and criminal injury and murder. This implies protection from breakdown of authority. Safety needs are expressed in a person's desire for a job with tenure and protection, an employment contract, desire for a saving's account, varying kinds of insurance, and a sound, reliable retirement plan. Safety needs dominate and are socially urgent in disasters, emergencies, during wars, disease and injury (particularly brain injury), crime waves, kidnapping, hostage holding, strikes, mass rallies, protests and marches, natural disasters, and breakdown of authority at the local, state, national or international levels. With any threat of chaos, human beings will regress from attempting to meet highest level needs to meeting the more powerful safety needs, belonging and love needs.[127]

Love and belonging needs emerge when physical and safety needs are reasonably gratified. These needs are expressed through a person's need for parents, a wife, husband, children, friends, colleagues, and acquaintances. The absence of these is keenly and deeply felt. A person strives for affectionate relationships, for a place within his culture, his group, his family. He will intensely strive to achieve these goals. Montagu's second category of nonvital human needs can be equated with love and belonging needs. He believes that if the person and the group are to survive, the need to be with others and the need for expression must be met. The fulfillment of these two needs is strategic if the person is to develop and maintain adequate mental health. The nonvital basic needs originate in the same kind of physiologic states as do the vital basic needs. Thus, the physiologic tension of the feeling of nondependency or aloneness leads to the need to be with others which, in turn, leads to the act of physical contact or association, which results in a feeling of security or interdependency. A person whose need for love and belonging is unmet feels lonely, separated, ostracized, rejected, friendless, abandoned, and restless. This need is thwarted for children (sometimes with disastrous personal results) when the family moves too often, or from the disorientation of the general overmobility brought on by technological advances and industrialization. It is also thwarted when one is without roots, or in a situation where one's roots or origin is despised, or cut off from one's family, friends, neighbors (such as often imposed through institutionalization, segregation in an intensive care or coronary care unit or communicable disease unit), or when one is a transient, an orphan, a foreigner, a displaced person, or a newcomer rather than a native.[128, 129]

Love and belonging needs are expressed through our desire for tenderness, affection, contact, intimacy, togetherness, and face-to-face encounter. They are expressed in the need to overcome feelings of alienation, aloneness, strangeness brought on by the scattering of family, friends, and significant others. Maslow and Montagu believe that the thwarting of love and belonging need satisfaction is the core reason for maladjustment and severe psychopathology. Maslow points out that love is not synonymous with sex, since sex may be viewed as strictly a physical need. In the true sense, sex behavior is multidetermined and multidimensional when viewed in relation to love and affection needs. Love needs involve both giving *and* receiving love.[130]

Esteem needs emerge with the fulfillment of love and belonging needs. A person has needs for a stable, firmly based wholesome evaluation of himself, for respect and esteem of self as well as esteem for others. There is a desire for strength, achievement, adequacy, mastery, and competence. There is a need for a feeling of confidence in the face of the world, for independence, for freedom. A person has a desire for reputation or prestige (esteem from others), status, fame, dominance, recognition, attention, dignity, and appreciation. Fulfillment of esteem needs results in self-confidence, feelings of worth, strength, capability, usefulness, adequacy, and a willingness to be a contributor to society. Need deprivation results in feelings of inferiority, helplessness, weakness, discouragement, and when serious, to compensatory and neurotic behavior. The respect sought by a person that results in a healthy self-esteem is the deserved respect from others rather than external fame, celebrity, and unwarranted flattery. Maslow states that it is helpful to distinguish actual competence and achievement that comes naturally and easily based on the person's inner nature, his constitution and biologic destiny from that based on sheer determination, will power, and responsibility alone.[131]

Self-actualization completes the hierarchy of needs, as designated by Maslow, and means that the person is self-fulfilled. As noted earlier, self-actualization is confined to adults. Young persons grow toward self-actualization. It is pointed out that even if all needs are satisfied, new discontent and restlessness soon develop unless the person is doing that which he is suited to do. A person must be true to his nature; he must be what he can be. He must fulfill his purpose in the world. A person has a desire for self-fulfillment. Self-actualization emerges after prior satisfaction of physical, safety, love, and esteem needs.[132]

From Montagu's point of view, all needs are dependent and must be satisfied by some object(s) in a manner in which they are structured. The requirements of these needs are such that they enjoin the manner in which they must be satisfied if the person is to function as a *healthy whole.* The facts of man's biologic nature—what man is—determine the direction that his development as a person must take. The biologic facts about a person give a biologic validation to the principles of cooperation or love in human life. In his view, the values for human life are biologically determined and are not matters of opinion. Acting against these inherent values disorders our lives as persons, as groups and as nations in the world of human beings.[133] Maslow sketches a profile of the self-actualized person as one who is

1. Healthy, polite, versatile, expressive, lets go when he wishes to, can drop controls, inhibitions, and defenses when deemed desirable, can relate interpersonally on a deeper level;
2. In control of himself and his impulses, can avoid hurting others, can have fun or give up fun;
3. Thinking of the present and the future, has a large array of responses and can move toward full humanness;
4. Efficient and superior in his perception of reality and his relations with reality, can see concealed or confused realities more swiftly and more accurately than others;
5. Superior in his ability to reason, to perceive truth, to make conclusions, to be logically and cognitively efficient, can discriminate between good and evil, means and ends;
6. Accepting of self, others, nature, is natural, simple, and spontaneous in his behavior;
7. Strongly focusing on problems outside himself, is not a problem to himself or generally concerned with himself, has a mission in life, a task to fulfill—some problem outside himself that uses his energies;
8. Displaying a quality of detachment, of a desire for privacy, autonomy, independence of the culture and the physical and social environment, has the capacity for fresh appreciation of the basic things of life, has a philosophical, nonhostile sense of humor;
9. Capable of intense peak or even mystic experiences (problem centering, intense concentration, self-forgetfulness, intense enjoyment of music, art, and sensations);
10. Able to feel an identification, sympathy, and affection for the human beings of the world (in spite of occasional anger, disgust or impatience), has a democratic character, and a desire to be of genuine help to the human beings of the world.[134]

Characteristics of basic or vital human needs demonstrate a fixed order in the hierarchy of needs and the existence of unconscious degrees of relative satisfaction of these needs. Each need represents but one functioning aspect of the whole person. There is a cultural specificity and generality of basic human needs. People in different cultures have more similarities than differences. Differences tend to be superficial rather than basic or vital and are more related to the individual's conscious motivational intent.[135] People have always met the demands of their basic needs and those needs derived from them by organization into cooperative groups, by artifacts, by the development of knowledge, values and ethics. "Man's institutions are based fundamentally on the satisfaction of his basic needs, though the structure of his institutions is made up of those derived needs which rise out of the cooperative process of satisfying the basic needs." [136] It is well known that persons in different human and cultural groups "learn to make the same responses to their basic needs in a large variety of ways." [137] Basic human needs cease to play an active determining role as soon as they are gratified, i.e., a basically satisfied person no longer has needs for air, food, safety, love, and esteem. Higher needs (after long gratification) may become independent of both their powerful prerequisites and their own proper satisfaction. For example, an adult whose love needs were satisfied in his early and past years becomes more independent than average with regard to safety, belonging, and love gratification in the present. It takes a strong, healthy, autonomous person to withstand the loss of love and popularity.[138] When a person has satisfied higher level needs and values, he becomes autonomous and is no longer dependent on lower need gratification.[139]

The arrangement of basic or vital human needs in a hierarchy is based on their state of power or strength. For example, safety needs are stronger than love needs because safety needs dominate in observable ways when thwarted; physical needs are stronger than safety and esteem needs. Additional conclusions regarding the hierarchy indicate that the higher the level of need, the more specifically human it is, the less imperative for survival, the longer gratification can be postponed, the easier it is for the need to disappear permanently, and the greater the survival and growth value for the person. When the person lives at the higher need level, there is greater biologic efficiency, greater longevity and health; thus pursuit and gratification represents growth toward health and away from psychopathology. More preconditions and greater complexity of life require more outside conditions for higher need fulfillment; in addition, the value that is placed on higher needs is greater than placed on lower needs by those gratified in both. Satisfaction of higher needs is closer to self-actualization than is lower need satisfaction.[140]

Human beings need love. Once satisfied, this person proceeds to develop in his own unique style, using these universal necessities to his own personal purpose. His development proceeds from within rather than from without toward self-fulfillment or self-actualization.[141]

Thus, through the use of the nursing process, the wholeness of man can be preserved. The framework presented based on human need theory provides the territory within which the nurse utilizes the nursing process—always focusing on safeguarding the unique wholeness of the person. The maintenance of the integrity of one's basic human needs is the responsibility of each person. The adult person in the parental or nurturing role fosters and facilitates the maintenance of basic human needs of the child. The nurse supports, fosters, facilitates, and intervenes with the well or ill client to maintain the integrity of the totality of these needs to assure an optimal level of wellness.

Summary

General systems theory has developed through the special attention it received in various areas of science and has contributed to the general framework within which natural phenomena are explained. System is seen as any recognizable delimited aggregate of interconnected dynamic elements that are in some way interdependent and continue to operate together according to certain laws to produce a characteristic total effect. It is concerned with activity and preserves a kind of integration and unity. A particular system can be recognized as distinct from others to which it may be dynamically related. Systems may be complex in that they may be composed of interdependent subsystems, each of which, although less autonomous than the entire aggregate, is fairly distinguishable in its operation.[142]

Systems are of two types—open and closed. A closed system is one in which no energy is received from an outside source and which does not provide energy to its surroundings. Open systems are those whose actions provide a continuous product output. The nature of the system is such that after any disturbance in input, its constant and time-independent characteristics may be restored, maintained, and/or reestablished. Although never in true equilibrium, the system maintains itself in a steady state, that is, neither static nor motionless. Instead it is marked by ceaseless activity and a change in the specific materials involved. The organism maintains its steady state by the fact that degradative processes in the cells are being continually compensated for by synthetic and anabolic processes. This work requires energy; therefore, the organism requires nourishment merely to exist—to maintain itself in a steady state quite apart from the energy that goes into effective work upon the environment. Open systems have the characteristic of equifinality, which is the ability to attain steady states independent of initial conditions. The growth or maturation of a living behaving system is an example.[143] Although the entropic process never becomes reversed and continues to some extent in all systems, in open systems a remarkable state of affairs occurs; for the time being and in certain parts or aspects of the system, entropy ceases (a measure of disorder). The measure or degree to which the system or part of the system stays away from entropy is called *negative entropy* (a measure of order).[144] Communication within the system is handled by a feedback mechanism that enhances its viability and its purposefulness. Decisions are an important component because of the selection choices and alternatives needed to maintain a steady state. Decision making, problem determination, and problem solving permeate life's activities and are significant to achieve the purposes of nursing. The nurse and the client as partners use the nursing process (a decision and problem-solving process) to achieve a state of optimal wellness.

If the system is a living behaving system, as it is in the case of a nurse and her client, communication within parts of and between the system and its environment is accomplished through perception. Perception, too, can be understood from a system point of view—at least in part—because input or messages are encoded, processed, and decoded with feedback adjustments so that awareness and adaptation to the environment are accomplished.

The territory within which nursing action takes place is basic human needs. These needs and their maintenance and integrity relate to physical, emotional, intellectual, social, cultural, and spiritual dimensions of man. They are vital to the development of man as a person, to the family, and to society. Human needs range from those that are life sustaining to those that enhance our living with ourselves and others.

Thus, the nurse, as a unique perceiving person in interaction with a client who is also a unique perceiving person, comprises that system of nursing whose goal is to meet the health care and nursing needs of citizens. Perceptions of both the nurse and client are fashioned from life experiences and knowledge, and each must be available (at least in part) to the other and communicated so that problems and needs related to health and its maintenance can be identified. The more information available, the greater the knowledge of alternatives, the keener the ability to predict outcome, the more effective the selection from alternatives, and the more successful the solution. The amount, quality, and focus of the nurse's knowledge and experience has an impact on the quality of her perception in a nursing situation. Similarly, the client's knowledge, experiences, and life style have an impact on how he thinks of his health, his predicament, and of the nurse as a helping person. The nursing process is designed to meet the client's basic human needs as these relate to health and nursing care. It is a data-gathering, decision process with a built-in feedback mechanism in the form of evaluation and modification. Thus, the nurse has the means with which to collect, designate meaning to, and make inferences about information, verify these inferences, plan to remedy designated problems or deficits, select the most appropriate alternative, and then implement this plan. Evaluation of the outcome, with modification, maintains the interaction in a viable state, and focuses efforts in the direction of a solution. This may result in reassessment, replacement, a change in implementation, then in reevaluation. The nursing process is cyclic. Using it in nursing practice is strategic to enhance the relevance and purpose of the nurse-client interaction.

In summary, the cyclic and parallel nature of the following theories as well as the nursing process itself are illustrated in this diagram:

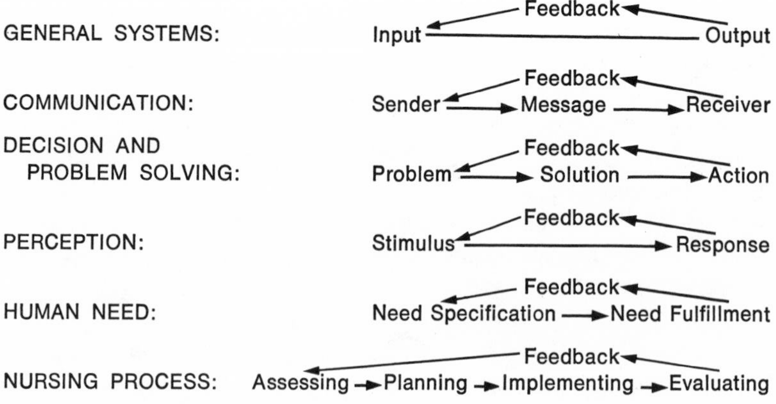

References

1. Banathy BH: Instructional Systems. Palo Alto, Calif, Fearon, 1968, pp 3–4
2. von Bertalanffy L: General System Theory. New York, Braziller, 1968, pp 37–38
3. Banathy, [1] pp 2–14
4. von Bertalanffy,[2] pp 142–143
5. Demerath NJ, Peterson R(eds): System, Change, and Conflict. New York, The Free Press, 1967, p 122
6. Hazzard M: An overview of systems theory. Nurs Clin N Am 26:391, September 1971
7. Simon H: The Sciences of the Artificial. Cambridge, MIT Press, 1969, p 52
8. Hazzard,[6] p 386
9. Raymond R: Communication, entropy, and life. In: Buckley W (ed): Modern Systems Research for the Behavioral Scientist. Chicago, Aldine, 1968, p 160
10. Mackay D: Informational analysis of questions and commands.[9] pp 204
11. Buckley W: Information, communication, and meaning.[9] p. 119
12. De Fleur M: Theories of Mass Communication. New York, McKay, 1966, pp 91–92
13. Rapaport A: The promise and pitfalls of information theory.[9] p 139
14. Schrödinger E: Order, disorder, and entropy.[9] pp 144–145
15. Rapaport,[13] p 139
16. Frick FC: The application of information theory in behavioral studies.[9] pp 182–183
17. Ackoff R: Towards a behavioral theory of communication.[9] p 216
18. DeFleur,[12] pp 91–93
19. *Ibid,* pp 93–94
20. Mackay,[10] p 206
21. Ackoff,[17] p 209
22. *Ibid,* p 213
23. Simon,[7] p 52
24. Griffiths D: Administration as decision-making. In Halpin A (ed): Administrative Theory in Education. London, Macmillan, 1958, Chap 6, p 140
25. *Ibid,* pp 131–140
26. Lee W: Decision Theory and Human Behavior. New York, Wiley, 1971, pp 8–9
27. *Ibid,* pp. 9–10
28. *Ibid,* p 10
29. Griffiths,[24] pp 131–140

30. Raiffa H: Decision Analysis. Reading, Mass, Addison-Wesley, 1970, pp ix–x
31. *Ibid,* p x
32. *Ibid,* p x
33. Newell A, Simon H: Human Problem Solving. Englewood Cliffs, NJ, Prentice-Hall, 1972, p 807
34. *Ibid,* pp 2, 9, 11
35. *Ibid,* p 53
36. *Ibid,* p 59
37. *Ibid,* p 59
38. *Ibid,* p 72
39. *Ibid,* pp 867–868
40. *Ibid,* p 809
41. *Ibid,* p 810
42. *Ibid,* p 860
43. *Ibid,* p 867
44. *Ibid,* p 826
45. *Ibid,* pp 847, 860
46. *Ibid,* p 55
47. *Ibid,* pp 56, 71
48. *Ibid,* pp 823–824
49. *Ibid,* pp 789–790
50. *Ibid,* p 790
51. *Ibid,* p 95
52. *Ibid,* p 91
53. *Ibid,* p 93
54. *Ibid,* p 88
55. *Ibid,* pp 88–89
56. *Ibid,* pp 92–94
57. Einstein A, Infeld L: The Evolution of Physics, New York, Simon & Schuster, 1938, pp 3–5
58. Raiffa,[30] p 220
59. *Ibid,* pp 240, 242–243
60. *Ibid,* p 243
61. Simon,[7] pp 55, 77
62. *Ibid,* pp 95–97
63. *Ibid,* p 112
64. Griffiths,[24] p 135
65. *Ibid,* pp 136–139
66. *Ibid,* p 140
67. *Ibid,* p 123
68. Rapaport A: Critiques of game theory.[9] pp 474–482
69. Buckley W: Society as a complex adaptive system.[9] p 490
70. Day RH: Perception. Dubuque, Iowa, Wm C Brown, 1966, p 42
71. *Ibid,* p 6
72. *Ibid,* pp 6–7

73. *Ibid*, pp 7–9
74. *Ibid*, p 42
75. *Ibid*, p 34
76. Vernon M: Perception through Experience. London, Methuen, 1970, p 1
77. *Ibid*, p 2
78. *Ibid*, p xi
79. *Ibid*, p 3
80. *Ibid*, pp 4–5
81. *Ibid*, p 5
82. *Ibid*, pp 6–7
83. *Ibid*, p 240
84. *Ibid*, p 239
85. *Ibid*, p 25
86. *Ibid*, p 25
87. *Ibid*, pp 25–26
88. *Ibid*, pp 25, 58
89. *Ibid*, p 59
90. *Ibid*, p 59
91. *Ibid*, pp 60, 67
92. *Ibid*, p 69
93. *Ibid*, p 99
94. *Ibid*, p 188
95. *Ibid*, pp 189–190
96. *Ibid*, p 191
97. *Ibid*, pp 196–197
98. Allport F: Theories of Perception and the Concept of Structure. New York, Wiley, 1955, pp 477–478
99. *Ibid*, pp 477–478
100. *Ibid*, p 485
101. *Ibid*, p 493
102. *Ibid*, p 526
103. *Ibid*, p 566
104. Maslow A: Motivation and Personality. New York, Harper & Row, 1970
105. Montagu A: The Direction of Human Development. New York, Hawthorn, 1970
106. Malinowski B: A Scientific Theory of Culture. Chapel Hill, North Carolina, Univ North Carolina Press, 1944
107. Kubie L: Instincts and homeostasis. Psychosom Med 10:15–30, 1948
108. Freeman GL: The Energetics of Human Behavior. Ithaca, NY, Cornell University Press, 1948
109. Linton R: The Cultural Background of the Personality. New York, Appleton-Century, 1945
110. Montagu,[105] p 113
111. Montagu A: On Being Human. New York, Hawthorn, 1966, p 49

112. Maslow,[104] p xxv
113. *Ibid,* p 2
114. Montagu,[105] p 117
115. Maslow,[104] p 20
116. *Ibid,* p 22
117. *Ibid,* pp 26, 28
118. *Ibid,* p 29
119. *Ibid,* pp 36–38
120. Montagu,[111] p 50
121. Maslow, [104] pp 36–37
122. Montagu,[111] pp 50–51
123. Maslow,[104] p 38
124. *Ibid,* p 39
125. Montagu,[105] p 117
126. Maslow, [104] pp 40–41
127. *Ibid,* p 41
128. *Ibid,* p 43
129. Montagu,[111] p 51
130. Maslow,[104] pp 44–45
131. *Ibid,* pp 45–46
132. *Ibid,* p 46
133. Montagu,[111] p 52
134. Maslow,[104] pp 137, 153–154, 159, 160–165, 168–171
135. *Ibid,* pp 51–57
136. Montagu,[105] p 133
137. *Ibid,* p 134
138. Maslow,[104] pp 57–58
139. *Ibid,* p 72
140. *Ibid,* pp 97–100
141. *Ibid,* p 135
142. Allport,[98] p 469
143. *Ibid,* pp 471–472
144. *Ibid,* p 475

Chapter Three •

Analysis of the Components of the Nursing Process

The maintenance of the integrity and the fulfillment of human needs to assure optimal wellness comprises the territory for nursing practice. Nursing is concerned with all of the biophysical, psychosocial, cultural, and religious needs of the client and fosters the meeting of these needs. When one or more needs are not met due to psychopathophysiology, immaturity, lack of knowledge, or lack of resources, it is the nurse who intervenes to offset the lack of need fulfillment as well as to assure the maintenance of the integrity of all other human needs of the client. Health colleagues may focus on selected unmet or partially met needs, designating the pathologic basis for the unmet status and prescribing medical or related therapies to eliminate or diminish the source of the problem. The nurse may refer selected unmet needs to appropriate health colleagues such as the physician, the clergyman, the social worker, or the dentist, and will collaborate with this person(s) as long as is needed. But the nurse views the client in his wholeness, as part of a family and a neighborhood, to assure that all needs continue to be met despite lack of fulfillment of one or more needs.

Thus, the nurse involves herself in preserving the wellness of the person and the well aspects of the ill person, continually seeking optimal enhancement of wellness and diminution of illness.

The nursing process is the designated series of actions intended to fulfill the purposes of nursing—to maintain the client's optimal wellness—and, if this state changes, to provide the amount and quality of nursing care his situation demands to direct him back to wellness. If wellness cannot be achieved, then the nursing process should contribute to the client's quality of life, maximizing his resources to achieve the highest quality of living possible for as long a time as possible.

Based on its theoretical framework, each component or phase of the nursing process will be developed and analyzed, according to the persons, both nurses and clients, involved in the process. The goal of analysis will be to suggest the components of the process appropriate to nursing actions, considering such factors as cultural background, age, level of wellness, degree of illness, as well as socioeconomic and educational levels. The unique aspect of each component as well as the interrelationships between components will be considered. The components of the nursing process follow a logical progression, but two or more may be operational at the same time. The time span for using the process will vary with the client's situation and may portray immediate and long-term goals.

The nurse and the client are viewed as partners in nursing, a subsystem of the health care system. Each person is viewed as a unique member of the family and the community—units of a social system. The nurse draws heavily on perception, communication, and decision-making in her use of the nursing process. The client utilizes these skills in his role by participating in assessing, planning, implementing, and evaluating his care.

The four phases, or components, of the nursing process used in this text are useful and inclusive. They incorporate many ideas stated by other authors who designate other, although similar, steps in the nursing process, the four components of which—assessing, planning, implementing, and evaluating—are the core of effective nurse actions. The nursing process is very vital and on-going, enhancing the level of success in solving client health and nursing care problems, utilizing the nurse's knowledge and skill to identify and solve client care problems, and solving them quickly, accurately, and economically. This implies a minimum waste of nursing personnel effort and facilities. The client gets the best care directly, in the shortest time possible, from the person who is best able to identify and solve his problem or problems.

The nursing process is systematized, appropriate for the well person or the family or for the acutely or chronically ill according to the situation. It can be used by nurse practitioners in whatever setting the client or family is in. It is important for the nurse to designate the client's wellness state as well as client problems, but it is just as important that she refrain from creating problems where none exist. Utilizing a logical, goal-directed process safeguards against creating problems. There is a cyclic nature to the nursing process, and the movement is constant between and among its components (Fig. 1).

The skills the nurse must have in order to use the nursing process are intellectual, interpersonal, and technical. Intellectual skills entail problem-solving, critical thinking, and making nursing judgments. Interpersonal skills are related to the ability to communicate, listen, and convey interest, compassion, knowledge, and information, and to obtain needed data in a manner that enhances

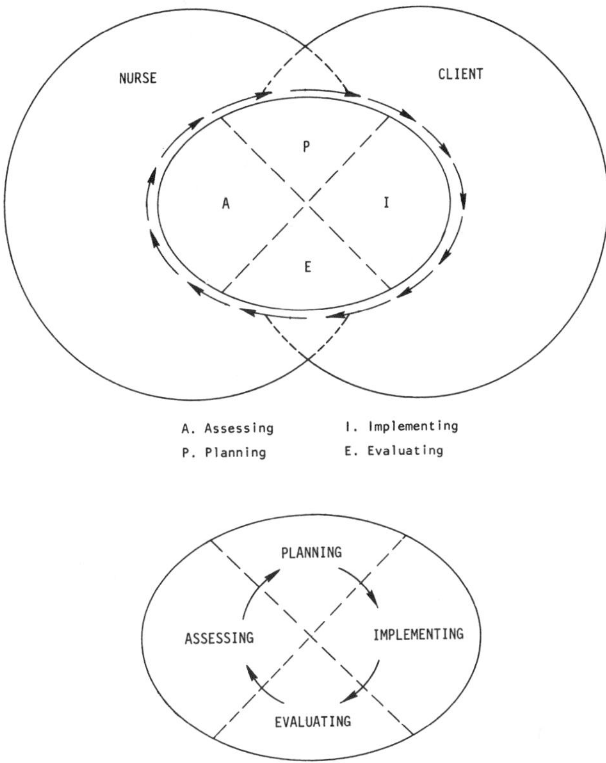

Figure 1.

the individuality of the client as a person. These skills foster relationships with the client, his family, co-workers, and colleagues. Technical skills relate to methods, procedures, and the use of equipment to collect data and to bring about specific results or the desired behavioral responses of the client. Decisions and decision-making are a part of every component.

Involvement in the nursing process assumes concern for persons, problems, places, and health. To engage successfully in this process, the nurse must be aware of the following pertinent premises.

1. A person is a human being endowed with worth and dignity.
2. A person has basic human needs that must be met.
3. Problems result when needs are partially met or unmet—due to limitations in physical, emotional, spiritual, social, and economic capability and the availability of resources.
4. Inability to fulfill one's basic human needs may entail the intervention of another individual who can help a person meet his needs or fill the needs directly until such a time as the person can resume that responsibility for himself.
5. A person or family presenting themselves for health care desires a client-centered approach that enhances their value and seeks solutions to their health and nursing care problems in the most effective, yet economic manner.
6. The nurse is interested in rendering high quality service to persons and families, no matter what their life style, economic status, or cultural or religious beliefs might be.
7. To utilize the nursing process and develop goal-directed nursing care plans the nurse must have up-to-date knowledge of theories from the physical, biologic, social, and behavioral sciences and must have mastered a knowledge of nursing as well.
8. The practice of nursing involves the ability to focus on another person and requires the full attention and energy of the nurse when she is engaged in the practice of nursing.
9. The heart of the nurse-client interaction is the development of a helping relationship in which the nurse fosters the client's personal development and growth by means of empathetic understanding, faith in the client's growth potential, respect and care for and about the client in an unconditional manner, willingly being available, and freely being one's genuine self.[1]
10. Successful nursing practice results from continued study—both formal and informal—and from an ongoing evaluation

of one's self-development and nursing practice, with plans to maximize strengths and minimize limitations.

11. The person or family demonstrate a willingness to share information, feelings, and concerns so that problems can be identified and solutions sought.
12. The nurse strives to realize her own self-development through the practice of nursing.
13. Every citizen has the right to quality health and nursing care rendered with interest, competence, and compassion.
14. Nurse practitioners need to focus on preventing disease, maintaining wellness, and rendering care to the sick.

Assessing

The assessment phase begins with the nursing history (including a health assessment) and ends with the verification of the wellness state or the designation of the nursing diagnosis or diagnoses. The purpose of this phase is to identify and obtain data about the client that will enable the nurse and/or the client or his family to designate problems relating to wellness and illness. If problems exist, then the first step toward a solution is to identify them.

The nurse's function is to assess wellness or illness and their extent. In the same instances, this ability may mean the difference between life or death for the client. In contrast to goals of other members of the health profession, the nurse involves herself with basic human needs that affect the *total* person rather than one aspect, one problem, or a limited segment of need fulfillment. The objective is to meet all basic human needs. The nurse will try to satisfy the needs of each person individually. Her effectiveness in assessing these needs depends on her knowledge of basic human needs, a solid base of anatomy and physiology, a knowledge of human behavior, major causes of morbidity and mortality, human growth and development, personality development, and knowledge of basic pathophysiology and psychopathology. A knowledge of various cultures with their beliefs and patterns, of major religions of the world and the obligations and patterns of the faithful following these religions, and of family and social organization and the economic patterns for that segment of society in which the nurse practices, as well as variations in other segments—state, regional, national, and international—are needed.

The nurse must first determine which needs are to be assessed, what and how much information will be needed, and from whom and where she can obtain this information or data.

Nursing care rendered in conjunction with the client or clients is directed toward maintaining a state of wellness, care of the sick, or both. Where wellness cannot be realized, supportive care is given so that the client can function to maximum capability.

It must be remembered that a need is not a problem in itself. The word *need* is used in many ways, sometimes as a noun and sometimes as a verb. It is used to denote a lack of something or to mean a requisite for bodily or psychic functioning. It is used frequently in everyday conversation. A need is not necessarily a problem, but a client can develop a problem when a basic human need is not met, or filled only partially. The terms *nursing need* and *nursing problem,* as heard in conversations and as they appear in the literature, refer to a nursing order, the action or intervention by a nurse to solve or resolve an assessed client problem. The word *need* denotes necessity or use for. The terms used in this text are *basic human need* and *client problem.*

The nurse may use a variety of theoretical models to designate basic human needs. Maslow's [2] Hierarchy of Needs, Montagu's [3] Vital and Non Vital Basic Needs, and Erikson's [4] Eight Ages of Man are both popular and useful models. The discussion of assessment will focus on these models. While categories of needs are general in nature, the nurse must assess individual or particular aspects of each.

Basic human needs refer to those that all people must satisfy to enhance their images of themselves as persons. The first category of needs, as distinguished by Maslow, are physiologic—food, oxygen, fluids, physical activity, rest, elimination, water, and sexual satisfaction. With the exception of sexual satisfaction, Montagu calls these vital human needs. All are present at birth except the need for sexual satisfaction, which differs because it is active only intermittently and can be satisfied by substitute measures. It is a need that must be satisfied by some persons if the group is to survive.

The second category comprises the need for safety and security, such as requirements for sameness, sureness, familiarity, and trustworthiness in people, things, places, and events. The third category is the need for love or belonging, including affection, warmth, kindness, and consideration in human relationships. The fourth is the need for self-esteem, such as respect, status, prestige, and a good reputation. For the child, these needs are met by parents or significant others by means of their approval and confidence in the child, their respect of him, and the fact that they regard him as a valuable person. The adult derives satisfaction from successful accomplishments in work and other activity. A sense of accomplishment carries with it feelings of adequacy, competency, and mastery. Needs for love and esteem form stepping stones to self-actualization, the fifth category. It is also viewed as the state of becoming, and involves the ability to control oneself, one's destiny, and one's needs rather than being controlled by them. Self-actualization is achieved in adulthood.

A person never outgrows his physiologic needs or his need for security, love, and esteem. Persons are motivated by all of these needs, but more so by some than by others at any given time. At times of stress, crisis, or illness, problems may arise in meeting some or all of these needs.[5] Illness does not mean these needs do not have to be satisfied; in fact, it may create heavier demands for fulfilling particular needs, the way in which they are met, or even by whom they would be met and when.

Physiologic needs must be met in preference to others only when the deprivation is life threatening. As soon as the threat diminishes, attention must be paid to other categories of needs. Factors that influence needs include age and sex; intellectual, emotional, educational, social, and financial capability; level of wellness or illness; type, location, and extent of pathophysiology and/or psychopathology; and the type, availability, and the effectiveness of the therapeutic regimen.

It is not possible to separate a person into his physical, psychologic, emotional, spiritual, educational, social, and cultural aspects. This is attempted academically, but in reality, a person is a unified entity. Rarely does a client have a physical problem that does not give rise to a psychologic component, a social and economic impact; likewise, a psychologic problem does not exist without a physical response to situations experienced. Need fulfillment is a motivating force. Needs motivate behavior directed toward achieving satisfaction, with each person meeting his particular needs in an individual manner.

By becoming aware of and by gaining knowledge about one's own inner experiences, a person develops a reliable basis from which the inner experience of others can be assessed. Within everyone, there is a basic drive for growth and development in the direction of optimal realization of his potential. His motivation and his perceptions are a trustworthy basis for action constructive for him. The nurse can facilitate and nourish the client's own basic drive for widening development. Any attempt to force this motivation into being or into activity will usually defeat its own purpose.

The client is responsible for himself. The nurse really cannot be responsible for him, although she is accountable and responsible for her own behavior toward him.[6]

To focus on one aspect, such as the physical, to the exclusion of the others, or to ignore the hypothesis that what affects any one aspect of an individual inevitably affects all other aspects, is to assess the client's problem in a limited manner. The limited perspective could create problems rather than diagnose or solve problems for the client.

Deprivations of needs, particularly those relating to food and oxygen, create a state within the person that demands satisfaction in order for the person to survive. The person will focus his behavior exclusively toward obtaining food or air. In *Man's Search for Meaning* the author, Viktor Frankl,[7] discussed the impact of hunger during wartime imprisonment and tells how prisoners dreamed of food, and of their exhaustive attempts to relieve their hunger. The fact that hunger is a total experience, not limited to a physical reaction alone, explains why some persons place a high priority on meeting basic life-sustaining needs. A starving person can hardly be expected to care for intellectual and interpersonal pursuits, economic advancement, and social status. Similar situations have been witnessed and experienced at times of natural disasters, such as floods, explosions, and other environmental upheavals. Once these needs are partially or completely satisfied, however, the person tries to fulfill other categories of his needs. By their reactions and behavior, people demonstrate their needs for safety and security, love or belonging, esteem, and, in the adult, self-fulfillment. The nurse has observed manifestations of low self-esteem, depression, withdrawal, hostile or aggressive behavior, and anxiety.

When considering the total person, it will be noted that he has needs in common with others. While these common needs are acknowledged, each person is still unique, whether he or she is a client or the nurse. The personality of every individual is unique; the combination of qualities and characteristics he possesses, his set of values, ways of reacting, interacting, and transacting can only be attributed to this one person alone. In some ways, his specific needs and reactions may have patterns similar to those of other persons, but each has some characteristic entirely different from that of any other person.

Another useful model is the eight stages of development toward maturity proposed by Erikson. Summarized briefly, these are:

1. *Basic Trust versus Basic Mistrust*: developing a sense of trust and security derived from affection and the gratification of

needs during infancy–from birth to 1 year of age. Hope is the outcome.

2. *Autonomy versus Shame and Doubt*: achieving a sense of autonomy in which the child views himself as an individual in his own right, beginning from his early childhood years (1 to 4 years old). Will power is the outcome.
3. *Initiative versus Guilt*: developing a sense of initiative, and a period of vigorous testing; imagination of adult behaviors occurs during the ages of 4 to 5. A sense of purpose is the outcome.
4. *Industry versus Inferiority*: developing a sense of industry and of duty and accomplishment, understanding real tasks; developing academic and social competence occurs during school age (years 6 to 11). Competence is the outcome.
5. *Identity versus Role Confusion*: A sense of identity, clarifying who one is and what one's role is, develops during the adolescent years (12 to 15). Fidelity is the outcome to be achieved.
6. *Intimacy versus Isolation*: A sense of intimacy, the ability to establish close personal relationships with members of both sexes begins to develop at the age of 15 years. Love is the lasting outcome.
7. *Generativity versus Stagnation*: Parental sense, productivity, and creativity for others as well as one's self; a sense of generativity develops during adulthood. Care is the outcome to be achieved.
8. *Ego Integrity versus Despair*: A sense of integrity, acceptance of the dominant ideals of one's culture, a sense of continuity with the past, present, and future, and the meaningfulness of life develops with adulthood and maturity. Wisdom is the outcome.[8]

The developmental stages of man provide a basis for understanding the client and a framework for determining wellness. The person must be viewed as a whole, with consideration given to his uniqueness, and the variation that characterizes his patterns of action, his view of himself, and his view of others. Going one step further, it would be useful to consider the unique characteristics of the client and nurse, rendering their interactions and their relationships also unique. Perhaps, this is what is "unique" about nursing. Paterson and Zderad explore these points further in describing authenticity with one's self. These authors believe that authenticity (self-in-touchness) is not only intellectual awareness of self but encompasses auditory, olfactory, oral, visual, tactile, kinesthetic, and visceral responses with each conveying unique meaning to man's consciousness.[9]

Inherent in the idea that each person is unique—demonstrating qualities, characteristics, needs common to other persons, and, at the same time, manifesting a particular difference, is to accept one's own individuality. The nurse must first understand her own strengths, her limitations, her pattern of response, her views, and her values, before she can be receptive to and accept those of her client. Her ability to assess and deal with her own behavior and that of the client presupposes a knowledge of human behavior and her belief in prevalent assumptions about behavior. Brown and Fowler compiled a useful list of these assumptions, which include a knowledge that:

1. A person's total response to a stimulus constitutes his behavior. The responses may generate from sources within or outside the individual—for example, a person who develops a fever in response to invasion by pneumococci or who shivers when he is in a cold room. Further, there is a covert as well as an overt aspect to each behavioral response. Covert responses include a person's thoughts, feelings, and motivations, whereas overt behaviors include verbalizations and human actions.
2. A person's behavior is governed by his available energy and is always within range of the maximum energy with which he is endowed. His behavior cannot manifest more energy than that which is available to him, although this quantity varies with his energy potential at any given time. Individuals differ from each other in their energy potential for behavior. Factors that might influence the availability of energy include caloric intake, metabolic rate, atmospheric conditions—humidity, temperature, barometric pressure, sensory deprivation or overload, age, sex, concept of self, timing and number of demands on the person at any given time, and his view of the value of these demands.
3. Behavior has a purpose, even though this purpose is not always obvious. The person may be trying to accomplish something. This accomplishment or lack of it may be in terms of gain, loss, or in maintaining one's self or situation.
4. A person's response to a particular situation is the best of that which he is capable of at a particular time. This does not preclude that the person can respond differently or more effectively by learning other patterns of response. These responses would be applicable to other client situations, partic-

ularly if there is some similarity between the situations. Knowing that a person is responding in the best way possible at a given moment makes it easier for the nurse to accept herself as well as the client as a person, whether or not she approves of a particular behavioral response.

5. A person's perception of what is happening to him has a greater influence on his behavior than what is actually happening or how it is interpreted by another person. The nurse must validate inferences about the client with him. The nurse's intentions and goals must be shared with the client and must be verified and accepted if her diagnoses and plans for action are to be successful.
6. Each person has a potential for striving forward. Since motivation to proceed in this direction is inherent within the person, efforts can be directed to stimulate and activate those forces having a positive influence. It may be necessary to designate basic human needs that must be fulfilled, whatever their category, as a precursor to meeting more mature needs. Efforts to stimulate advancement must be based on an accurate assessment of the current status of the person's needs, which will serve as a baseline in evaluating change and the direction of change.
7. A person satisfies most of his needs in an interpersonal manner with other persons and/or groups of persons, each demonstrating dependent, independent, and interdependent behavior. The quality and quantity of these manifestations change as the person progresses from infancy to adulthood. Their quality increases as each person experiences and copes with human situations as he strives for self-fulfillment or self-actualization.[10]

The nurse, as the helping person, must be willing to understand the client from his own frame of reference. She senses and seeks to understand what is real and meaningful to him at any point in time and must know how he sees things, or feels about himself. She is sensitive to his conscious feelings and the meanings underlying his outward communication. The nurse maintains a clear distinction between meaning that originates in herself and that which originates in her client. She attempts to understand his meaning at a particular moment with the idea that this understanding is subject to correction and change as new data become available.[11] Caring for and about the client is unqualified; that is, no conditions are attached to it. The client does not need to earn approval or liking by expressing some desires and suppressing others, by portraying certain attitudes or beliefs and denying others, or by being one type of person and not another. This rules out the need to label clients as *uncooperative-cooperative, demanding-docile,* etc.[12] These beliefs are conveyed to the client during all phases of the nursing process. Efforts to establish a helping relationship begin with the first nurse-client interaction, at the time the client enters the health care system, and it continues as long as this interaction is needed.

In addition to knowledge of basic human needs, assumptions about human behavior, and characteristics of a helping relationship, the nurse needs a strong knowledge of anatomy and physiology, chemistry, physics, microbiology, psychology, sociology, human growth and development, mathematics, literature, art, philosophy, pathophysiology, psychopathology, and theology. The content of these courses provides the basis for her knowledge of man in his world, of the person who is well (including her own self-development), and, in addition, provides a basis for recognizing a change in a person's state of wellness. The selection of specific principles from these biologic, physical, and behavioral sciences provides the rationale for the nurse's actions, facilitates her decision making, and enhances her person-centered interactions. Specifically, basic principles and theories from selected biologic, physical, and behavioral sciences will provide the framework for assessing the client's health status and his need for nursing intervention.

A framework of factors to be assessed will focus on those common to all persons. The nurse must adapt and adjust this framework to incorporate specifics that determine the unique aspects of a particular person and/or family. The collection of data related to these factors will also be devised creatively by the nurse to suit settings in which she is functioning. For example, factors for assessment may have dimensions different for the school nurse, the office nurse, the nurse in the community health center, the nurse in a health maintenance organization, the nurse in a nursing home, the nurse in a rural setting, an urban setting, in an acute care setting or chronic care setting, or the nurse working with persons of a particular age group, such as infants, adolescents, or the elderly, with men or women, or with those who are sightless, deaf, or mentally retarded. Initially the nurse starts with a prescribed list of factors, but she should exercise her intellect and creativity in developing an in-depth list, based on her observations, experiences, and an analysis of factors portrayed by clients with similar problems.

Among these factors are those relating to age, sex, education, growth and development, socioeconomic, cultural and religious elements, biologic and physical status, emotional status, coping patterns, interactional patterns, life styles, employment, the client's view of health and illness as it relates to himself and his family.[13-15] In addition, consideration must be given to the client's expectations of health care and his awareness of the roles of the health care practitioners, particularly of the nurse; the physical, social, emotional, and ecological environment in which he lives and works; and the human and material resources available and accessible to him.

When assessing factors related to age the nurse should know the needs, roles, expectations, and behaviors relative to infancy, childhood, adolescence, adulthood, and senesence for male and female persons. Maslow's Hierarchy of Needs,[16] Montagu's Vital and Nonvital Basic Needs,[17] Erikson's Eight Ages of Man,[18] and Duvall's Family Development [19] are useful guides to the collection of meaningful data and provide a basis for validating inferences and designating problems. Age and sex are extremely important factors when considering a person, whether he or she is the client or the nurse. These factors are combined with all others and influence each other significantly.

When assessing factors relating to the needs of persons from different racial groups, the nurse needs to know their customs, rites, rituals, traditions, expectations, and views, including their implications for wellness, for the sick role, for suffering, illness, dying, and death.

When assessing the needs of persons from different nationalities and from varying geographic and climatic areas the nurse needs to know the customs, rites, rituals, traditions, roles, and expectations of persons living in that country as they relate to wellness and illness. She needs to consider the geographic and climatic experiences of the person, as well as his environmental adaptability when assessing his needs.

When assessing religious factors, the nurse must know the various religions of this era as well as the beliefs, rites, and rituals of each. A knowledge of the rules (with implications) freeing individuals from participating in religious rites and rituals because of illness or handicap, of the rites and rituals of the different religions, as they apply or are available to the sick, disabled, the suffering, the dying, and to the person who has died, is necessary.

A person's formal or informal education, acquired through experience, must be considered. Included in this factor would be an investigation into any specialized language used by the client during education or employment. Specialized interpretations or uses of words and phrases or of foreign words or phrases are important to know. For example, the nurse needs to know how the 2-year-old shows that he needs to urinate or defecate. Failure to understand his communication of these needs may create a problem for the child where none existed before. This is particularly significant when the child is away from the home setting—as in a child health clinic, a day care center, or a pediatric unit of a general hospital. Another important facet of the educational factor is to assess the client's problem-solving ability.

As to socioeconomic status, it is important to assess the client's perception of his status. The perception and expectation of clients with varied socioeconomic backgrounds—from the deprived to the wealthy—must be considered. The impact of the client's job on his perception of himself as well as on the needs fulfilled by his job must be determined.

The assessment of growth and development should be broadened to include physical, social, intellectual, and personality elements in establishing growth and development patterns. Age, sex, and culture are inextricably bound to growth and development and may be assessed simultaneously.

To assess biologic, physical, and emotional status, the nurse needs a model of wellness to serve as a base. The model must incorporate such factors as age, sex, socioeconomic status, and culture. Models of wellness may differ for different age groups, for men and women, and for persons from varied socioeconomic and cultural backgrounds. Knowing what is expected or normal for bodily and psychic functions provides the framework within which the status of each can be assessed for a person or a family. The nurse must know what constitutes normal nutrition, fluid and electrolyte balance, oxygen demand, elimination of wastes, rest and sleep activity, hygiene, circulation, comfort (freedom from pain and discomfort), recreation and diversion, and sensory integrity.

This knowledge gives the nurse a broad framework within which to work, but is of minimal value until she assesses the normal variation for each subfactor for a specific person. When additional data are forthcoming about this person, judgments are made from these initial data. For example: if a person's blood pressure is 110/80 mm Hg, it may be considered normal. However, it may also be a sign of organic disorder in an aged person who normally has a blood pressure of 150/90 mm Hg. A clear picture of what is normal for each particular person is of primary importance.

The nurse must have a knowledge of major pathologic and psychopathologic insults to the human person at various age levels, for each sex, for the major racial and cultural groups, and of those prevalent in specific geographic areas or in a certain environment. For example, structural abnormalities, malnutrition, infections, cancer, and accidents are major problems among infants and young children; for the preschooler, communicable diseases, dental caries, schizophrenia, retardation, speech defects, leukemia, and kidney infections must be considered. The older child, the adolescent, and the young adult are prone to accidents, respiratory conditions, allergies, cancer, obesity, suicide, schizophrenia, communicable diseases, behavioral problems, such as faulty eating and sleep patterns, interpersonal maladjustment speech disorders, learning difficulties, and acne. As a person advances in age, conditions causing illness and death become more numerous. Major disabilities are related to cardiovascular-renal disease, cancer, diabetes, pneumonia and respiratory impairments, suicide, and accidents.

With a knowledge of normal human function and a working knowledge of major psychopathologic and pathophysiologic insults, symptoms of onset, causes, patterns of treatment, and outcomes, the nurse is prepared to begin the assessment phase of the nursing process. She must focus on prevention, as well as care of the sick, and rehabilitation. She continually increases her knowledge of wellness, of alterations from wellness, symptom manifestation, treatment, human reactions to illness, and qualities of coping ability, by evaluating her own actions and studying the assessment and analysis of problems presented by persons with a major disability.

When assessing a person's interactional patterns and his ability to cope with his problems, the nurse determines ways and means available to him should a crisis or stressful situation arise. Coping patterns vary greatly among individuals and within family groups. The number of variables that constitute a stress situation may determine a person's ability to cope successfully with a problem. This ability may differ from time to time and is influenced by his view as to what constitutes a stressful situation. In family settings, the ability to cope with a problem or problems may be pooled and some of the detrimental effects of a stressful situation may be offset by the strengths of individuals in the family. Interactional ability may bear on how, when, and in what manner particular basic human needs are met. This is especially true for such needs as safety, love, and esteem. It can also be true for physical needs and for adult self-fulfillment.

Considering the person's life style, his expectation of health care, his view of his own health and/or illness, and what he expects of health practitioners, and the availability and accessibility of human, health, and material resources, may help to determine whether he presents himself for a health status evaluation or for the diagnosis and correction of a health problem, or if therapy that is instituted will, in fact, be successful. One's life style, including the environment in which one lives and works, cannot be separated from the person if that person is to be viewed in his entirety. Failure to consider a person's life style constitutes one of the many affronts to personalization rampant in the health care system. This failure may create problems where none existed, or it may create an atmosphere wherein therapy will not be helpful. The following example will support the nurse's need to determine life-style factors, if the assessment is to designate correct and useful action.

• *Situation Report*

Mr. Strong, a 70-year-old gentleman with swollen ankles, pain in his legs, and difficulty in breathing was admitted to a health care facility for diagnosis and treatment. A plan of nursing care was to be developed. This was his first hospitalization and his first evening was described as uneventful. He was given a sedative and hypnotic at 8:30 P.M. At 1:30 A.M., the night nurse found him walking in the hall. She intended to escort him to his room, but as she approached to take his arm, he became frightened, and quickly struck out and hit her on the lip with his hand. She became frightened; the night supervisor was called and arranged to have the night nurse's bruised lip treated. She then summoned the security guard, who found the patient, frightened and confused, hiding in the bathroom. He was put to bed, and the following morning the day nurse found him awake, upset, and worried. He told her that he thought he hit a nurse but wasn't sure.

During the period of care, the nurse found one bit of information about this elderly gentleman that had not been known to nursing personnel, or if it had been, was not considered important or useful. The patient had been a night watchman for 40 years up to the day of his admission. His sleep-awake pattern was therefore different from that prevailing in the health care facility. He had worked alone, policing the halls and rooms of the building at which he had been employed. He had to be on the alert so as to protect himself against intruders. Sharing this information with the nursing staff made quite an impact. The nursing care plan that subsequently evolved included efforts to help the patient reverse his day-night pattern while he was hospitalized. He was helped to stay awake for longer periods during the day. His medication for sleep was changed and given to him at midnight. Having this information on the day of admission, giving it value, and incorporating it into the nursing care plan might have spared the patient and night nurse an unpleasant experience and the negative feelings that arose from it.

Nursing History and Health Assessment

A nursing history is taken to obtain needed data systematically, through a planned interview with a client. The collection of this information, the analysis of data, designation of problems for nursing intervention, and the implementation and evaluation of this plan are the responsibility of the professional nurse. A specific time must be designated to obtain the history, and the place where it is to be taken—an inner city clinic, the client's home, a hospital room, a physician's office, an industrial camp or community mental health center—should afford privacy. The history should be taken as soon as the nurse and the client confront each other. The time spent should be adequate to obtain as much information as possible in an unhurried manner. Time should be given to impart information to the client. An interview guide developed by the nurse, or by a committee of nurses, may be used initially. A number of authors have developed nursing history guides that could be useful to the beginner.[20-23] Some of these guides lend themselves to inpatient interviews whereas others can be adapted for the outpatient. The format of the interview should vary according to the setting and services rendered and to the functions of the nurse. Although core data about the client as a person will always be needed, specific areas of information will differ if the nurse is admitting a woman in labor, if the client is being admitted into the health care system, or if the client is being interviewed in a self-care unit, a long-term care facility, or in his home.

In some instances, checklists and questionnaires have been devised for the convenience of the staff and to save time. Often these can be used routinely and contribute a negative factor because only items on the form are used. Some are merely filled out and filed away with no use made of obtained data. At times, it may be appropriate for the client to fill out information sheets. This, of course, is only appropriate if the client can read and write and if he is oriented, aware, and has the strength to do so. In any case, an interview with the nurse should verify, clarify, and yield additional information deemed necessary. The interview gives the nurse the opportunity to see the person and to use her perceptual abilities not only to obtain information but to communicate her concern, interest, and willingness to understand. It gives her the opportunity to reinforce those behaviors conducive to wellness.

The nurse should strive to develop her own format, which should allow for flexibility and adaptability with persons having a variety of problems. Eventually a specific guide may no longer be necessary. The nurse will focus on general and specific topics, making adjustments as they are needed, to obtain the data she needs to assess the client's health status and delineate his problems accurately. While the data are being collected, the nurse validates inferences to assure accuracy in interpretation. When the nurse infers the existence of a problem, or assumes a condition from known facts or evidences, she should confirm or validate the problem, condition or situation with the client. Making inferences about information and validating them with the client emphasizes the nurse's desire to get an accurate picture of the client's experience and will minimize the possibility of imposing a judgment based on inadequate information, a few symptoms, or a limited social history. This will also protect the client from becoming the recipient of stereotypes, prejudices, or generalizations held by the nurse.

The time involved in obtaining a nursing history is well spent; it may be a significant factor in saving time in any services or care rendered to the client. Failure to obtain data about the client before problems are assumed or solutions imposed may be more time consuming, may drain the physical and emotional energy of the nurse as well as the client, and create a climate of mistrust and insecurity for him. It would add considerably to the cost of his care.

During the interview, the nurse should seek to clarify points that are not understood. She should allow the client to express himself completely and obtain a clear picture of his expectations. Should he be unable to express his needs because he is too young, too old, too sick, unconscious, or is in a life-threatening situation, a person who knows the client well should supply available information. All efforts should be made to involve the client as soon as possible and as much as possible. For example, as soon as the life-threatening situation has eased, the client should participate as much as possible. This holds true for all clients who are unable to participate temporarily or who can participate partially or only on a nonverbal level. The nurse will use her own senses to collect information as well as to consult with family members, neighbors, co-workers, and other health team members during the interim in which the client cannot participate. As soon as possible, the nurse will continue with the nursing history.

Up to this point, verbal interaction between nurse and client has been emphasized. The nurse uses various communication techniques as open-end questions, and/or reflection, to facilitate communication. The selection of techniques and their appropriate use is based on how they are used and if they facilitate exchange of data. A technique is not good or bad within itself. How appropriately it has been used and the outcome will designate its value. The nurse and client have picked up nonverbal cues that must be clarified and verified.

In conjunction with the nursing history, the nurse performs a health examination. A health examination includes the collection of data relating to physical, psychologic, and emotional dimensions of the person, his family, and his neighborhood, with the nurse fully utilizing her senses of sight, hearing, touch, and smell as well as any data-gathering tools available to provide needed information. Limiting the examination to the physical dimension alone fails to provide data that reflect the wholeness of the person. Many authors have contributed via text and audiovisual media to the technique of physical examination. No attempt will be made to duplicate this information here. The text book by Samuels and Bennett, *The Well Body Book*,[24] demands particular attention, for it contains a wealth of health information, including how to do your own physical examination. The nurse can hardly utilize less information than is readily available to the public as she assesses the health-illness status of the client and his family.

The nurse exercises her perceptual and judgmental skills to note the client's posture, facial expression, manner of dress, physical limitations such as the failure to use a hand, an arm, or a leg, to note deformities, an absence of parts, such as teeth or extremities, the presence of scars, discolorations, cuts, and the use of eyeglasses, contact lenses, hearing appliances, crutches, and canes. The nurse uses sight, hearing, touch, and smell to collect these and other data. (See Appendix B for a list of observations that can be made using sight, hearing, smell, and touch.) Critical judgments are made about a selected datum, clusters of data, the relationship and interrelationship of selected data and clusters of data as well as the absence of data.

While sight and hearing are used extensively throughout the

interaction, touch can elicit data about skin temperature, muscle tension, moisture, variation in strength of extremities, swellings and masses, palpable distortions in configuration, areas of pain and tenderness, and tremors. The nurse's sense of smell can supply data relative to usual and unusual odors, pinpoint specific breath odors, such as tobacco, alcohol, mustiness, sweetness, use of chemicals—commercial mouth washes and agents that are unknown or not easily recognizable, smells that denote one's pattern of living or job, smells of wounds, particularly those infected or with decomposed or dead tissue, odors of bodily excretory products—urine, feces, vomitus, sweat, and such odors as perfumes, medicines, liniments, and salves.

The nurse will measure bodily function, using palpation, observation, and measuring tools, such as thermometer, stethoscope, or sphygmomanometer, to obtain readings of body temperature, heart rate, quality and characteristics, respiratory rate, and blood pressure. Specimens such as urine, stools, vomitus, sputum, and secretions from other bodily parts or draining wounds may be collected. Some tests can be done immediately, using chemical tapes and kits. Others must be sent to the laboratory for analysis.

The nurse could assign supportive health and nursing personnel, qualified to collect specimens and proceed with analyses, to assemble these laboratory data.

When the client feels he has had an opportunity to express his feelings, concerns, goals, desires, and expectations, and the nurse has affirmed and validated any inferences and there are no gaps in the information she needs to make a nursing diagnosis, the interview can be terminated. At this point the client can be told how these data will be used as well as the plan for continuing the interaction into the planning, implementing, and evaluating phases. The client should have felt that the nurse was interested in him as a person and that she had conveyed in her communication—both verbal and nonverbal—that she viewed him with respect and dignity. The fact that she called him by name, listened with full attention, anticipated his questions, and spoke with him rather than to him, conveys respect. She will have refrained from using language unfamiliar to him and guarded against responding to his questions in a condescending manner. If his condition was critical, with life-threatening respiratory or circulatory problems, she participated in relieving the crisis and then focused immediately on his participation. She was also attentive to the desires and concerns of persons important to the client.

During this interview and performance of the health assessment, the nurse and client begin a relationship based on trust, respect, concern, and interest. The client should feel that the nurse is truly interested in him as a person, that she is concerned about his welfare, and that she recognizes and respects him as a co-partner, designating and meeting his needs for health and nursing care. The client knows that he not only is viewed as a valued person, but as a member of a family or group of significant others, and a member of a neighborhood and a community.

When this nursing history interview is terminated, the client should know who the nurse is; who will be responsible for his care; that some one person knows his views, his fears, his concerns, and his expectations; that someone knows the basic human needs that he fulfills himself and those he cannot fulfill. He knows how to summon the nurse, where she will be, when and how he can communicate with her, and when she will see him again. If he is an inpatient in a health care facility, orientation to the environment and available services may be included in the interview. The nurse may consider it prudent to delegate this orientation to another member of the nursing team.

After the data are collected, the nurse seeks additional relevant data from family members, from persons accompanying the client, or from persons in the household. Other members of the health and nursing teams, significant members of the community, and available records and reports are also used to obtain data.

The nurse sorts, organizes, groups, categorizes, compares, analyzes and synthesizes the data about the client obtained up to this point. Decision making and judgment are inherent in every phase of the nursing process and are particularly significant during assessment. The nurse decides what to ask, when to ask it, and how to ask it. She decides when to listen, how to listen, and how long to listen. She uses judgment throughout the interview by focusing on some areas in depth and by passing more briefly over others. She judges when there may be more to the meaning of a topic than that which the client has told her. She summarizes all available data, then makes one or more of the following judgments:

1. No problem exists and the client's state of wellness is affirmed. A plan to maintain wellness is developed with the client that the client then implements. Periodic reassessment of wellness will be made, and the client will present himself for these at given intervals. The client will seek reassessment sooner if he suspects a problem.
2. No problem exists, but there is a potential problem that may

be offset by giving the client information on prevention and planning for a future interview with him. It may be necessary to refer the client to another health care member.

3. A problem exists but is being handled successfully by the client and/or his family. Plans for periodic reassessment will be formulated, but the client will return for these at non-scheduled times if he thinks it necessary. The problem may be new or it may be a long-standing one. Pharmacologic and mechanical aids may be used to resolve the problem, for example, medications, crutches, hearing aids, colostomy and ileostomy appliances, and prostheses.
4. A problem exists that the client needs help in handling. Providing this assistance—whether it is information, environmental, caring, socioeconomic, pharmacologic, and/or mechanical, will either resolve the problem or make it easier for the client and/or family or neighbors to handle it. Appropriate provision, including referrals to health team members and social agencies, will be planned with the client. The client, nurse, and other health team members share in implementing the plans. Implementation continues until evaluation indicates that the problem has been resolved or has decreased or reassessment deems a change in plans is necessary.
5. A problem exists that the client cannot handle at this time and its nature prevents family and neighbors from helping him to resolve it. Health care intervention is needed. Specific members of the health care team such as the physician, nurse, dentist, psychiatrist, physiotherapist, or nutritionist may be assigned to help the client. With health care intervention (one or more members), the problem can be specifically diagnosed, treated, and resolved. An example of such a situation is dental caries.
6. A problem exists that must be studied further and diagnosed to resolve or to keep it within manageable proportions. Ambulatory and/or inpatient health and nursing services may be needed. The problem may be solved completely; for example, a foreign body or obstruction of some kind is removed. In other situations, an elevated blood sugar may be diagnosed, treated, and provisions then made for continued management on an ambulatory service.
7. A problem exists that is not incapacitating to the client at present, but its resolution requires intervention that would

render the client dependent for a specific period or indefinitely. Surgical interventions and certain medical regimens are examples. Inpatient care is generally necessary. A specific medical diagnosis may have been made before the initial nurse-client interaction. Acute care followed by extended care and/or ambulatory care may be part of the planning.

8. A problem exists that places heavy demands on the client's ability to cope with it and that the family cannot resolve; they could, however, contribute emotional support and money for intervention by members of the health care and/or nursing team. These problems may be life threatening; for example, myocardial infarction, cerebrovascular accident, diabetic acidosis, cirrhosis of the liver, bleeding peptic ulcer, drug addiction, and depression. Immediate and continued intervention by members of the health care team, on an inpatient basis, is required.
9. A problem is imposed unexpectedly on the client or his family because of an accident, injury, or natural disaster, or is self-imposed (attempted suicide). The problem may or may not be a threat to life. If it is life threatening, health team members must attend to it immediately to reduce the crisis situation, if possible. If not, the crisis imposes problems on family members. If the crisis is resolved or the situation is more incapacitating than life threatening, situations discussed in items 1 to 8 may prevail. An example would be the child who is found to have an obstruction in the respiratory tract. Removing the obstruction—a bottle top, balloon—quickly and effectively relieves the problem, with no residual disability. If the problem cannot be resolved, immediate surgical intervention may be required. When the crisis is due to a natural disaster, like flood, in which food, water, and shelter become unavailable, although the lack of these can be tolerated for some time, illness is a direct result of such deprivation; with survival threatened as the time without these necessities lengthens.
10. Problems exist that are long-term and permanent. The client is able to cope with some but not all of his problems, and other persons, such as family, nursing and health team members, clergy, lawyer, or social workers, may have to intervene to cope with the problem and provide care on a continuing basis. Long-term health and nursing care must be provided within the home, community health center, community men-

tal health center, an extended care facility, or a combination of these. An example would be the person with a congenital anomalie as spina bifida.

Any one, or any combination, of these situations may exist for a client at one point in time, but he may experience any number of these situations in his progress to wellness. The nurse then, as noted above, designates specific problems stemming from the larger problem area.

Nursing Diagnosis

The nurse concludes the assessment phase with a nursing diagnosis.[25-28] This diagnosis specifically indicates that: (a) no problems exist that demand the intervention of the nurse or another member of the health team, or (b) the precise identification of all problems that had to be resolved so that the client could experience the wellness optimum for him. Problems will be stated in terms of client problems, and result when basic human needs are either not met or are met inadequately.

Making a nursing diagnosis requires a high level of intellectual skills. It is the most strategic aspect of the nursing process and concludes the assessment component. Without a nursing diagnosis there is no reason to continue to other components of the process in an effort to solve a client's problem. There will be no basis for planning or intervention or any basis for evaluative judgments about this client's problems.

Considerable work has been accomplished related to nursing diagnosis. A most notable recent development had been made by the National Conferences on the Classification of Nursing Diagnoses, initially sponsored by the St. Louis University School of Nursing and Allied Health Professions nursing faculty and co-chaired and coordinated by Kristine Gebbie and Mary Ann Lavin. This is an historically significant development. It gives appropriate recognition to the importance of the nursing diagnosis and provides a method for pooling the knowledge about nursing diagnosis. While no one classification system has emerged, we believe that basic human needs can serve as the rightful framework for the categorization of nursing diagnoses. A quick glance at the nursing diagnoses assembled to date allows the viewer to designate easily the human need to which the nursing diagnoses refers or for which the nursing diagnosis serves as the label for a deprivation or alteration in meeting the need. In other words, the client has a problem when one or more of his human needs are unmet or poorly met or excessively met. This client problem is the nursing diagnosis.

A nursing diagnosis may be further qualified by delineating additional problems stemming from the original diagnosis, by prefixing the diagnosis with such adjectives as acute, chronic, full, complete, partial, or minimal to mention a few. In addition, following the diagnosis with "due to" gives the psychopathophysical, social, cultural, educational, developmental, economic or environmental reason for the lack of need fulfillment. This "due to" will facilitate the selection of nursing strategies to offset the need deprivation.

For example, sleep is a human need. Sleep patterns have been described quantitatively and qualitatively in the literature. In addition, the pattern for a specific person can be designated. To follow the pattern and then awake refreshed to accomplish the tasks of the day would be the expectation. Lack of fulfillment or failure to meet this need would be designated as sleep deprivation, excessive sleep, or disturbed sleep. Sleep deprivation may be acute, chronic, occasional, or sporadic. It could be due to a noisy environment, excessive use of caffeine, failure to allow time for sleep, fear of dark, to brain neoplasm, to continued disturbance resulting from medical therapy (as in an intensive care unit), or to the onset of disease yet undiagnosed.

A nursing diagnosis may be singular or diagnoses may be numerous depending on the health status and deprivations or alterations in meeting needs of the client. Nursing diagnoses may cluster in relation to a human need. They may include sleep deprivation, sensory overload, sensory deprivation, body image distortion, immobility, oxygen and carbon dioxide alteration, pain, low self-concept, or distortion of cerebration, to mention a few. Thus, the meeting of the human need with diminution of the client problem is the goal. The planning to diminish the problem, then application of the prescribed strategy and evaluation of the achievement of this goal will follow the making of the nursing diagnosis. The determination that the human need is met is the object for the evaluation phase of the nursing process.

Planning

The planning phase begins with the nursing diagnosis. During this phase plans are made with the client and his family to deal with his problems, as diagnoses. It is expected that the goal or outcome desired will be the resolution of the problem diagnosed, i.e., human need fulfillment. For example, if sensory deprivation is the problem, then sensory integrity will be the goal. All efforts will be exerted to achieve this goal or outcome. Precise problem identification with specific actions planned to achieve the outcome will provide the framework and data for the evaluation phase of the nursing process.

The purposes of the planning phase are: (a) to assign priority to the problems diagnosed; (b) to differentiate problems that could be resolved by nursing intervention, those that could be handled by the client and/or members of the family, and those that had to be referred to other members of the health team or handled in conjunction with health team members; (c) to designate specific actions, and the immediate, intermediate, and long-term goals of these actions, as well as expected behavioral outcomes for the client; and (d) to write the problems, action, and expected outcomes on the nursing care plan. The planning phase terminates with the development of the nursing care plan, which is the blueprint for action, providing direction for implementing the plan and providing the framework for evaluation.

If no problem exists and the nurse verifies the client's state of wellness, a plan for periodic reevaluation of the client's state of wellness is formulated jointly. Plans to continue wholesome living patterns will be reinforced, and specific information the client requests or needs will be given, such as immunization, accident prevention, and poison control information. Brochures may support and reinforce or expand the information. The client is requested to return immediately if symptoms appear or if he feels he has a problem. Thus in her interaction with the well client, the nurse participates with him in the assessing and planning phases, but the implementation and evaluation phases are the client's responsibility.

Ordering or Priority Setting

If specific client problems are diagnosed, effort is exerted to assign priority to each. The nurse uses her own judgment and considers the client's views in assigning priorities. During ordering or priority setting problems can be conveniently classified as high, medium, or low priority. As high priority problems are resolved fully or in part, the order in which remaining problems are resolved may have to be reevaluated. Problems in the medium- or low-priority category may be given a higher rating at some time. The more life threatening the problem is, the higher the priority assigned. A number of problems may be considered high-priority simultaneously, such as an obstructed airway, ineffective breathing, impaired circulation, or gross hemorrhage. It could be assumed that the nurse and the client and/or his family would generally agree about giving life-threatening problems a high priority.

Each client problem should be classified so that the integrity and unity of the human person is maintained. Again, Maslow's hierarchy can be useful in designating priority, with physical problems given priority over safety needs, then needs for love, esteem, and self-actualization. Although physical needs take precedence, as soon as problems that stem from an inability to meet basic human needs at this level are diminished, high priority must be transferred to problems that arise because basic human needs in other categories have not been satisfied effectively. In some nursing situations, there may be no problems with physical needs initially, and high priority is given to needs for self-esteem. For example, the client who has a poor opinion of himself may disregard safety measures and refuse to eat. Resolving the problem with self-esteem may also solve problems in other categories that stem from the original problem area.

In all situations, the client should be closely involved in decisions that set levels of priority or order. In instances in which the nurse and the client assign different priorities to the same problem, the difference can be resolved by mutual communication of the reasons for setting a particular priority. Priorities set by the client should be considered.

Other factors that influence priorities as set for the client include the availability of personnel and resources, the cost of needed services, and the approximate time needed to resolve his problem or problems, particularly from his point of view.

Once priorities have been identified by the client and the nurse, an ordering of these priorities is established. The nurse designates possible solutions for each problem diagnosed, but solutions offered by the client should be included. The possible success of each solution to a problem is estimated, based on scientific principles and/or sound research. Variables such as age, sex, life style, education, socioeconomic, and cultural background of the client, his ability to cope with his problems, and his physiologic and emotional status, as they relate and effect suggested solutions, should be considered. The nurse predicts, as accurately as possible, the consequences of each solution. Then, in cooperation with the client, she selects the solution most likely to be successful in resolving or diminishing his problem. If the client endorses the solution, his efforts and cooperation in implementing that solution will insure its success.

The solution may be multifaceted, with immediate, intermedate, and long-range implications. An immediate goal is one that can be accomplished within a short span of time. An intermediate goal can be attained over a period of time—teaching, supporting, preventing acute problems—whereas a long-range goal is oriented toward the future. Goals for the client include preventive and rehabilitative aspects as well as crisis or immediate aspects relative to his present wellness-illness status. For example, if the client's problem is constipation and this difficulty has been a long-standing one enhanced by the frequent use of laxatives and self-administered enemas, to relieve the condition temporarily would neither resolve the problem nor provide long-term benefits. The client may experience immediate relief, but requires sustained relief if an impact is to be made on the problem and if discomfort, inconvenience, and the cost of relief measures are to decrease. Although the solution may be to relieve the constipation, the actions instituted may have an immediate effect—to give immediate relief by using pharmacologic or mechanical agents. Additional actions may have intermediate and long-range goals, such as developing a regimen to increase fluid intake, increase fruits and vegetables in the diet, plan specific time for defecation, and provide privacy and an unhurried atmosphere, while enemas and laxatives are gradually withdrawn. This regimen would be instituted after pathologic conditions that cause constipation, such as strictures, tumors, and congenital anomalies, have been ruled out. Thus, to relieve constipation for the present would not have a lasting impact on the problem, causing the client to return repeatedly to obtain relief.

Intermediate and long-range goals that stem from solutions to the problems will be concerned with preventing complications, rehabilitation, and health instruction. Continuity of care is enhanced by this farsightedness, and the cost of health care, both in time and money, to the client and to health personnel will be considerably less. Immediate, intermediate, and long-range goals of the solutions are appropriate if the problem can be resolved and in those situations in which the problem will continue. Long-range goals may focus on preventing additional problems or on preventing intensification of the present problem. This would be true, for example, when the problem is permanent blindness. Failure to designate long-term goals may mean the difference between a client who can become maximally independent as he strives toward the optimal degree of wellness for his particular problem or a client who remains dependent and therefore derives only limited joy from living because of multiple complications and problems.

When a problem that can be resolved by nursing intervention has been identified and the best solution has been selected based on the strengths and resources of the client and/or his family, the availability and competency of nursing and health personnel, and the resources available for health and nursing care, specific actions and expected outcomes for the client's problems must be designated.[29]

Problems that can be resolved by nursing intervention must be differentiated from those that require not only the attention of a nurse but also that of one or more members of the health team, such as a physician, physical therapist, or clinical pharmacist, and problems that can best be resolved by other members of the health team or by specific members of the community. Problems relating to spiritual or legal matters—a will, housing, job—should be referred to the appropriate person or agency. A well-designated and developed referral system should be established so that appropriate persons can be involved with a minimal loss in time, and maximum use be made of persons and agencies qualified to solve various client problems. Methods and forms are generally available for use by agency health care personnel.

Nursing Orders or Nursing Strategies

The solution to any one problem may be an adaptation of a known solution or it may be designed specifically for that problem. When the solution most likely to be successful is selected, specific nurse actions designed to achieve the short-term, intermediate, and long-range goals of that solution must be delineated. These actions are also called *nursing orders* or *nursing strategies.* Nursing actions must be clear, purposeful, moral, capable of being accomplished, and adapted to the particular life situation, beliefs, and expectations of the client. Because nursing action is designed to solve the problem, the outcomes expected as a result of that action should be stated in terms of the client's behavior. Only by specifying and recording the client's behaviors can the nurse judge the impact of her action. Statements of nurse behaviors can be a basis for evaluating the nurse's competency, but if the effectiveness of the care rendered is to be evaluated, expected outcomes must be stated in terms of client behaviors.

In some health care settings, established policy may dictate the kind of action to be implemented and the person who will implement that action. Policies pertaining to nursing care should be formulated with nursing personnel. Health team members may develop policies and procedures for handling particular problems or governing some particular area in a health care facility. Policies bypass thinking; the person involved in implementing a policy must know the specific circumstances under which it applies. When the situation is recognized, the policy is applied. Policies may vary from one designating the number of visitors per hospitalized client to established policies and procedures formulated in the event of cardiac arrest. They appear to be more numerous in settings where personnel tend to be less prepared. Thus, there are policies to safeguard clients. For example, a policy stating that every hospitalized client 65 years of age or over must have side rails on his bed probably resulted from evidence that older clients often fall from their beds during their periods of hospitalization. This policy does not protect the 50-year-old with an orientation or behavior pattern that might result in a fall. Nursing judgment is needed to interpret policies and make appropriate adaptations in the best interest of the client. Policies and procedures need to be reviewed from time to time. Circumstances under which they were formulated may no longer exist and other policies may be needed. The nurse must be informed of prevailing policies, for and by whom they were instituted, of the allowable latitude in their interpretation, and what procedures must be followed to change the policy. The nurse is obligated to bring to the attention of appropriate persons policies potentially detrimental to clients or those which are misinterpreted or overly implemented by personnel. Clear, precise policies and procedures developed for units such as coronary care, kidney dialysis, or intensive care help these facilities function quickly and smoothly. These policies should also be reviewed periodically, particularly if clients demonstrate high levels of anxiety, signs of sensory overload, or sensory or sleep deprivation. Precise data to support any request for a policy change that would improve care and enhance the individuality of the client would be helpful. All policies should be expressed in writing and dated to safeguard the nurse against pressures that perpetuate patterns of action that are custom rather than policy.

The quality and quantity of nursing actions delineated to solve a client problem and effect a specific behavioral change will be determined by the nurse's knowledge and experience. Her knowledge of biologic, physical, and behavioral sciences as well as her nursing knowledge, clinical experience, and knowledge of resources—persons, books, her ability to seek out consultation from other nurses or health team members—broadens the options, variations in actions, and the application and expectations from the actions. The nurse designates actions that will most likely effect a behavioral change and that have been approved by the client. Documenting these nurse actions—what should be done, when, and how—constitutes nursing orders or nursing strategies.

When actions are designated for problems, according to priority or ordering, a decision is made as to who will carry out these actions, when, and how. The nurse may select those she will do for and with the client, those the client can perform for himself or that can be performed by his family with or without supervision, and those actions that can be accomplished by certain members of the nursing team. To assign the nurse who is best able to perform the nursing actions—making adaptations and modifications to suit the client, his strengths, limitations, level of wellness, illness, and personal preferences—a team conference may be appropriate for planning. It not only serves to orient nursing team members involved in the care of the client but may also be useful to insure that the client's interests and preferences will be considered, his basic human needs met, and his problem solved.

It must be obvious to the reader that both the assessment and the planning phases draw heavily on intellectual skills—critical thinking, decision making, judgment, observation—and interpersonal skills. The latter are used to establish rapport through verbal and nonverbal communication, including active attentive listening. Technical skills are used mainly in the assessment phase, but to a lesser extent than are intellectual and interpersonal skills. Intellectual and interpersonal skills are paramount in the planning phase.

During the entire planning phase, activity is directed toward the quality and quantity of nurse actions that will be needed to resolve or minimize problems. This activity effects specified behavioral change within the context of immediate, intermediate, and long-term goals, and culminates in the formulation of the nursing care plan.

Nursing Care Plan

The nursing care plan includes precise data about a specific client. These data are organized in a systematic, concise manner that facilitates overall nursing and medical goals. It clearly communicates the nature of the client's problems and the nature and relationship of related nursing and medical orders. It contains all information about the client, his preferences, his problems and the priorities assigned to each, problems and complications to be prevented, and expected outcomes with prescribed nursing actions.

The format for the nursing care plan should flow from the goals set. Space should be provided to designate client problems, solutions, nurse actions. and expected outcomes. The health care agency may have a nursing care plan form. If none is available, a nursing care plan form can be developed that would be appropriate to clients and to problems that are most likely to be seen in the health care facility. Or, the plan may be developed and included as part of the problem-oriented system that may be utilized by multi-disciplinary health personnel whose focus is the resolving of client problems relating to health-illness (nursing as well as medical, dental, dietary, etc.).[30] A number of authors have contributed substantially to nursing care plans and nursing care planning.[31–35]

A well-written nursing care plan provides a central source of information about the client, with a description of his problems and a plan of action to solve them. A nursing care plan has become increasingly important with the increased number of professional and nonprofessional personnel involved in the nursing and health related services rendered to the client.

The plan is developed by the professional nurse who obtained the data for the nursing history and performed the health examination; she is most knowledgeable about the client and has the data needed for planning effective nursing care. The plan she develops incorporates elements in the medical care plan so that designated regimens complement rather than conflict with each other. When the most knowledgeable person creates the nursing care plan, recognition of the client's individuality is most likely to be enhanced. She is the one who is most likely to know the client's ability to cope with situations; thus, intervention will not be planned where none is needed and at those times when the client is coping with his problems satisfactorily. The client's right to appropriate independence, as well as to interdependence and dependence in the management of his wellness and illness is fostered.

Once the nursing care plan is developed, it can be utilized as a separate entity or included as a component part of the prevailing system utilized in the health care agency, provided this system is truly client focused and problem-oriented.

The development of the nursing plan is, therefore, a knowledgeable, creative, and intellectual activity and should be so designed as to mark its identity explicity, even if the client's name is omitted. When one nurse is responsible for developing and keeping the plan viable, additional data about the client obtained by other nursing and health care personnel can be directed to her. Often, important data are lost or given low priority when they are submitted to the wrong person, or the receiver places little value on the information because she has no knowledge of the client's problems or his goals or does not view the datum in relation to other available client data.

A clearly stated nursing care plan is the most effective means of assuring the client that his problems will be solved and his basic human needs fulfilled. Problems created by failing to realize some basic human need and by using verbal statements or nonverbal gestures that are depersonalizing or lower the client's self-esteem could be minimized. The drain on the time and energy of nursing personnel and the frustration and anxiety experienced by the client when he senses that the staff is not interested in him or is unaware of his needs and his preferences can be problem-solved. If the client knows the nurse is interested in him, if he knows what to expect and who to summon, he is likely to be more relaxed and less anxious. He also is less likely to make frequent requests for errands or small duties—often only to assure himself that someone cares and knows that he exists. If the client's problems, his preferences, and his life style are known, the actions of the nursing staff will be more useful and purposeful. Time wasted through ineffective or multiple actions by many nursing personnel, because goals are lacking, communication is poor, and facts about the client are not being used properly, could be reduced substantially.

The time used in preparing a nursing history and health assessment, a nursing diagnosis, and a nursing care plan that includes writing orders is time well spent. Failure to take the time to assess and plan before intervening contributes to the misuse of time and wasted efforts and talents of nursing and health care personnel. The cost in economic, physical, and emotional terms can hardly be estimated. Economically and morally, the profession of nursing cannot permit this misuse of human and material resources.

Two client-nurse situations that will help to focus on these points follow:

• *Situation One*

Mrs. Weak, a 48-year-old woman who was discharged after a two-week period of hospitalization was referred to a community health nurse. The referral stated that Mrs. Weak had had gallbladder surgery. Her medical diagnosis was terminal carcinoma, primary site, the gallbladder. The nurse went to the client's home to evaluate the situation; actually she should have gone to assess the client situation. Perhaps she was influenced by the fact that Mrs. Weak was terminally ill. When she went to the home and found the woman seated alone in the living room, the nurse could only recommend that she seek admission to a nursing home. The nurse was informed that Mrs. Weak's husband had been taken to the hospital with chest pain the day she was discharged. The nurse did not feel it was safe for this woman to be alone. Mrs. Weak firmly refused to consider the nursing home, and the nurse's anxiety about her mounted. When the nurse returned to the community agency, she expressed her concern to her supervisor, who helped her by logically delineating the data in the situation so that a more accurate judgment could be made about Mrs. Weak being alone. To her surprise, the nurse did not know whether Mrs. Weak could walk, care for herself, or what assistance from family and neighbors, if any, was available to her. Did Mrs. Weak know how to summon help for herself in case of an emergency? After a thorough assessment, it was found that Mrs. Weak could manage very well by herself and actually had little disability, considering that she had a terminal illness. An effective assessment preceded the development of a plan of care acceptable to Mrs. Weak. It was realistic and focused on the wellness she experienced as well as on her illness.

In another situation, automatic actions based on a specific condition rather than on the condition within the context of the client's total situation caused the client to refuse nursing care.

• *Situation Two*

Mrs. Wise was a 40-year-old woman who was admitted with a diagnosis of anemia. She was ambulatory, and the medical plan was designed to find the cause and type of anemia as well as to determine appropriate treatment. Mrs. Wise was a career woman who had a responsible job. While assisting with the physical examination on the day Mrs. Wise was admitted to the health care facility, the nurse noted that the client had a colostomy. Without obtaining further information from Mrs. Wise, the nurse planned to irrigate the colostomy the following day. She attempted to do so, but Mrs. Wise promptly and clearly refused her help. The nurse felt that the client had rejected her, for she thought she was being helpful. She had overlooked the fact that Mrs. Wise had had the colostomy for

> 14 years and had established effective regulation without irrigation, with minimal care, and without assistance. Also, during these 14 years, Mrs. Wise had never disclosed to anyone but her husband that she had a colostomy. Had the nurse assessed the client's problem and taken a nursing history, she would not have been rejected and would have used her time and energy more purposefully, directing her actions to include the problem that brought the client to the health care facility—anemia.

Planning has two additional dimensions, horizontal and vertical. Horizontal planning has been discussed up to this point as problem—solution—goals (immediate, intermediate, long-range)—nurse actions. The additional dimension involves vertical planning, which fosters the logical progression of nurse actions and has its greatest impact when the nurse and client interact on a continuing basis throughout a 24-hour-period. Vertical planning includes timing specific actions, paying special attention to basic human needs and the client's circadian rhythms. For example, if the nurse is required to perform numerous actions and there are accompanying actions by other members of the health team, such as a physical therapist, occupational therapist, medical technologist, or physician, actions should be planned to permit undisturbed periods of sleep and undisturbed meals. Not to include these considerations during the planning phase may cause problems for the client and divert some of the energy he needs to cope with the task at hand away from fostering an improved state of health. Thus, the time factor is a major consideration in planning. It involves not only the amount of time required for and when nursing actions will take place, but the biologic timing of the client, which must be known and preserved. Luce has contributed valuable information concerning biologic rhythms that has direct bearing on the nurse's understanding of herself and the meeting of human needs.[36]

Once developed, the nursing care plan is implemented. At this point, the plan should not be considered a finished product. It is merely a guide to actions and must be kept viable by additions and changes based on the client's problems, on resolution of these problems, and on continuous collection of data as nurse and client get to know and trust each other.

The format of the nursing care plan should be such that it is easy to use and contains enough space to record everything that needs to be written down. Although brevity and clarity are characteristics of a useful nursing care plan, its use will be diminished considerably if brevity becomes the exclusive goal. The development of the nursing care plan is the nurse's privilege and is, in fact, a creative, purposeful, intellectual activity. It is an expression of a nurse's knowledge, her ability, and her focus on the client. It will also serve as the model for all actions initiated by other members of the nursing team. Thus, the nurse contributes to the effectiveness and goal-direction of others—all of which benefits the client.

Every effort should be made to develop a method of displaying and storing the nursing care plan so that it is readily available to the nurse when she needs it. No one should have to wait to review the plan because someone else is using the folder that contains it. Space should be provided so that changes and dates can be filled in without erasing. For study and research, the nursing care plan and information about how it evolved should be preserved, since it contains first-hand data about persons, their problems, solutions to these problems, and goals that may be useful in developing a nursing science.

It is interesting to note that Bertha Harmer made similar statements in 1926 in her book *Methods and Principles of Teaching the Principles and Practice of Nursing*. She suggested that nurses develop a written program of nursing care and that these programs be kept and filed under a classification of diseases. She believed that nurses would collect a mass of information about nursing specific persons and about nursing in general. Organized knowledge would be available in a form that permits the nurse to go back and check her work, to note progress in content and method and ". . . to compare facts presented for the study of a great many cases of the same class, and of different classes, and to select facts common to all cases of the same class; in other words, to formulate principles, to organize knowledge—the process of making knowledge, which is science."[37]

Also, the plan can be used as a model for the care of other persons with similar problems, with a similar ability to cope with problems, or it can serve as a point of self-improvement for the nurse as well as for all members of the nursing team.

Sharing the nursing care plan with nursing and appropriate health team members fosters a better understanding of the client, and the efforts of all health and nursing personnel are more likely to complement each other. Each team member will find that she can function in her role more effectively and successfully when the roles of her associates are clarified. Health team members should be encouraged to utilize the nursing care plan as a resource. In situations where a joint plan of care is formulated by the interdisciplinary health team, the nursing care plan will be incorporated into the joint plan. Nursing diagnoses and specifically determined nursing strategies should be clearly visible in the joint plan or problem-oriented system.

The planning phase ends when the nursing care plan has been designed and developed. This plan is an effective medium for transmitting information for planned care in that all team members can accurately perceive and implement the care intended. It should be designed so that it can be utilized quickly and results in nurse actions that are meaningful and directed toward resolving the client's problems.

In some situations, client problems, particularly those that are critical in nature, may be preplanned for use within the framework of the nursing process. Preplanning involves the use of nursing or problem-solving processes to develop plans of action when time is important and life may depend on a predetermined plan of action. An example of such preplanning would be actions to be taken in case of fire. Available data about fires, how they start, various types of fires, combatting various types of fires—electrical, chemical, etc., about combustibility of materials, level of vulnerability of a particular setting, fire regulations, materials available to extinguish fires, techniques for safety of personnel and clients, and methods of prevention should be sought. In addition to literature and manuals, a specialist in fire fighting should be sought for consultation. A plan could be drawn up by nursing and health team members, clients, and other interested persons, then tested for accuracy and efficiency—including dissemination of the plan, instructing personnel about their roles, and testing equipment. A periodic review to reinforce the plan should be scheduled. Thus, as soon as the nurse assesses the fire, the plan indicated by the situation is implemented. The applicability and effectiveness of the plan can only be evaluated after it has been used. Preplanning may include all members of the nursing team in a particular setting, health team members, and citizens. Other situations in which preplanning is valuable include such crises as cardiac arrest, mass disasters, such as floods and earthquakes, drownings, explosions, emergency treatment for accidents (poisonings, burns). The more intense the crisis and the greater the immediate threat to life, the less time there is for thinking and problem-solving and therefore the more important preplanning becomes. The plan is revised as new knowledge of how different crises should be handled becomes known. Thus, there is less time between the assessment and the implementation phases. When the crisis has passed or diminished, the usual problem-solving methods prevail.

In addition to preplanning by health and nursing team members and citizens, the nurse may find it necessary to preplan a selected number of problems to enhance the safety, security, and life of the client, and which could be used until the problem is relieved or its intensity and immediacy diminishes. For example, if the nurse is working in a school setting and among the students there are a few with epilepsy, she may preplan the care they should receive for a seizure. This preplanning involves collecting a great deal of data about the client's pattern and manifestation of convulsions; the presence or absence of an aura; the client's method of handling himself before the onset; the characteristics and effects of the convulsion; data from the literature about convulsive seizures; identifying problems associated with convulsive seizures (falls); known methods of promoting safety and minimizing injury during or after a seizure; identifying persons likely to be involved, such as teachers and classmates; ramifications for the client when a seizure occurs during a swim class, in the science laboratory, or in the lecture hall; formulating a plan of action in the event of a seizure and communicating that plan among teachers, friends, the client, or selected classmates who may become involved. Suggestions shared by these persons should be incorporated into the plan. Once the plan is implemented, it should be evaluated. Other plans might be devised by the nurse as she needs them; for example, what to do in the event of sudden death (in whatever setting this may occur), choking, obstructed airway, and hemorrhage, to mention a few.

Preplanning may be appropriate for anticipated crises and problems, where thinking and planning time is limited and where immediate action is necessary to enhance the client's safety. Preplanning focuses on an event and is often heavily technical. Continued preplanning beyond the selected crisis, for more than "just in case," or outside the framework of the nursing care plan defeats its purpose. Preplanning should be used within the various phases of the nursing process, and incorporated into a client-centered, goal-directed framework. Excessive, exclusive, or inappropriate use may be dehumanizing and depersonalizing, focusing on an event or problem rather than on the client, or focusing on one problem to the exclusion of others. It can add a measure of confidence to the nurse and security for the client if she knows what to do in an emergency. Preplanning may be strategic in that it may help the nurse to prevent a situation, and the plans should be shared with nursing and health team members, family members, and the client, if appropriate.

Implementing

Once the nursing care plan has been developed, the implementation phase begins. Depending on the nature of the problem and the condition, ability, and resources of the client as well as the nature of the action planned, the client or his family, the nurse and client, the nurse alone, or nursing team members who are to act and function under the nurse's supervision may implement the nursing plan. Implementation may also be accomplished by the nurse, assisted by nursing team members, or in cooperation with health team members. Any combination of or all of these situations may prevail. In other words, in any one situation, some planned actions may be accomplished by the client, some by the nurse, and others by nursing team members. In other instances, only the client may be involved. This is particularly true if the client is well and prevention is the goal. The client may be able to continue wholesome health practices or new health practices in place of faulty ones. Some or many care measures may also be performed by the client's family, not only for clients who are homebound, but also for inpatients in health care facilities.

The implementation phase of the nursing process draws heavily on the intellectual, interpersonal, and technical skills of the nurse. Decision making, observation, and communication are significant skills, enhancing the success of action. These skills are utilized with the client, the nurse, nursing team members, and health team members. While the focus is action, this action is intellectual, interpersonal, and technical in nature.

With the nursing care plan as the blueprint and immediate, intermediate, and long-range goals firmly in focus, actions are put into practice. During this phase, the viability of the nursing care plan is tested. The plan is not carried out blindly; all thinking and decision making have been completed during the two previous phases.

The nurse continues to collect data about the client as a person, his condition, his problems, his reactions, and his feelings. Additional information continues to be gleaned from other nursing and health care personnel, and from family, neighbors, teachers, and records.

The success or failure of the nursing care plan depends on the nurse's intellectual, interpersonal, and technical abilities. This includes her ability to judge the value of new data that become available to her during implementation, and her innovative and creative ability in making adaptations to compensate for unique characteristics—physical, emotional, cultural, and spiritual—that become known to her during her interaction with the client. She must have the ability to react to verbal and nonverbal cues, validating inferences based on observation. Paramount during the interaction is her acceptance of herself as a person, and confidence in her ability to perform the independent nursing functions inherent in the planned action, recognizing those that are interdependent and in which she contributes to fulfilling the medical care plan. She must have a realistic understanding of herself, recognizing and accepting her strengths and limitations; be convinced of her own personal worth and find meaning in her life; meet her own basic human needs reasonably well, so that she can, with willingness and joy, give of herself to another—her strength, her courage, her faith in the competency of the client, her value for life, her knowledge, her skill, and her time during the interim when these might be needed by another. She must feel comfortable being herself—authentically herself. She needs to feel secure and adequate in her relations with others. If her needs are satisfied and she can control her own thoughts, feelings, and actions, then she will be able to focus on the thoughts, feelings, and needs of another in a wholesome comfortable manner. Although the nurse meets many of her needs outside the nurse-client interaction, her needs for recognition, monetary compensation, creative expression, and self-fulfillment are satisfied in her function as nurse through her interactions with clients, their families, co-workers, and colleagues.

The more wholesome her view of herself as a person and the stronger her philosophy of life, the less likely the client will experience depersonalizing encounters with the nurse.

The following situation, as told by Nurse B, illustrates an inadequate and inappropriate interaction during the implementation phase:

> When 65-year-old Mrs. Brave was admitted to the hospital on an ambulance litter, it was evident that she needed an admission bath. I, Nurse B, was asked to help Nurse A. Mrs. Brave moaned but did not talk. She lay in the fetal position, on her right side. She could not or would not change her position. Nurse A reacted roughly, making comments about how dirty

> the patient's family was. The poor lady, I am almost positive, must have heard what Nurse A was saying. At this point I believe Mrs. Brave was frightened and, perhaps angry, so that she became increasingly uncooperative. I tried to talk to Mrs. Brave to reassure her that she had nothing to fear from me and that I was not going to be unnecessarily rough with her. I said nothing about her odor; Nurse A referred to it almost constantly. I tried to encourage Mrs. Brave to help with the bath and extend her extremities. With two nurses attending her, it must have been very confusing to Mrs. Brave; she did not know how to or to whom she should respond. Nurse A did not cover her very well while bathing her, and as I tried to cover Mrs. Brave she grabbed the covering and drew it tightly about her. Apparently Mrs. Brave had been sick for a while at home and had no one to care for her except her husband.

The nurse should feel confident, comfortable, and satisfied in relating to clients. If she does so, she will not use the client, her co-workers and colleagues, or the setting to satisfy her own personal needs. The assessment and planning phases require these same qualities in the nurse; in addition, the implementation phase tests her endurance, her love, her intellectual ability, and her interpersonal and technical skills.

The amount of time spent with the client varies significantly, ranging from a short to a prolonged interaction. This encounter could range from minutes and hours per day to daily, weekly, monthly, or yearly continuation of the relationship; the interaction may be continuing or intermittent. Interaction should be planned precisely by the nurse and client, with allowances made for the unexpected.

It is strategic that each interaction be goal-directed and purposeful. An atmosphere of intellectual and interpersonal "thereness" should prevail. In other words, the interaction demands alert, observant, and attentive behavior by the nurse. In this atmosphere, the nurse conveys her concern for the client, and her interest in helping him achieve the wellness optimum for himself. In her manner of speech, her tone of voice, her gestures and mannerisms, she imparts her views of this person as one who has dignity and value. This means conveying dignity and value even though the client may not feel, look, or smell good, or if he acts, looks, or thinks differently from other persons.

In the client's presence, the nurse uses her perceptual skills to their fullest. As she looks at the client, maintaining eye contact as much as is comfortable, she observes his situation—his posture, appearence, and actions, his immediate environment, and the presence of other persons. She may initiate conversation or allow the client to do so. The client is given the opportunity to direct the conversation and initiate topics of interest to him. The nurse actively listens to what he is saying, indicating by nods or short statements that she understands. She asks for clarification if she does not understand and helps the client focus on a topic if he has difficulty doing so. She adjusts and adapts her manner and the content of her communication with the client when the situation is such that verbal expression is difficult, temporarily not possible (client has a tracheostomy), or is permanently impossible. The nurse must be able to judge when it is necessary to listen more patiently, when an interpreter is needed, when mechanical devices such as paper and pencil are needed, and when hand signals can be used. The nurse and the client will also need to know when verbal communication is not necessary, silence is appropriate, touch is useful and appropriate, as well as when and where it should not be used, or when words are conveying a message different from the nonverbal message coming through. The nurse judges how to word her statements and questions in a manner that will elicit responses within the client's capabilities (physical, emotional, social, educational), and uses repetition, as needed, without demeaning or demoralizing the client. If the nurse cannot understand the client's message, she freely admits this and seeks ways or persons who could enhance her understanding.

The nurse is fully aware of the need to communicate with the client who does not respond in the usual and expected manner. Talking to the infant or to the comatose or unconscious client is important, not only from the standpoint of conveying a message, but in order to maintain as much sensory integrity and contact as possible. The verbal as well as the accompanying nonverbal message may be received, even though the receiver is unable to return verbal messages. The nurse can meet needs for safety, security, love, and esteem by talking to the client, by her manner, or her voice, particularly if she holds the client's hand, feels his brow, or supports a shoulder. Further, very young or very old clients who are isolated, or who become disoriented, may feel alone or abandoned if human contacts are limited or task-centered. It is extremely important to prevent sensory deprivation for these clients.

The nurse may find that the client needs her full attention and she will choose to sit with him in full view, yet with the privacy of their interaction protected. At other times, she may find that opportunity for conversation will be available while bathing or feeding the client. Since the nurse has considerable data about the person, she will be able to use it to explore or suggest topics. She may plan a caring activity, using this activity as a vehicle to foster conversation. The nurse will judge when technical activity will enhance the client's safety and security more than verbal assurances. Thus, by viewing action in terms of the goals of nursing care, based on client problems, the nurse's focus on achieving a goal is facilitated, often meeting needs on several levels simultaneously by a particular action. For example, relieving dyspnea has physical as well as emotional implications for the client. If the nurse does not perceive or respond to the client's dyspneic state his anxiety may increase, adding additional stress to his respiratory reserve.

When the purpose of the nurse-client interaction is to perform a technical action, the success of the nurse's activity can be heightened if she focuses on the recipient's immediate needs as well as on the technical procedure itself. The client is entitled to an explanation of the action, his role and expected behavior during the action, the expected results of the action, the type of equipment, solution, etc., the discomforts to be anticipated, the position to be maintained, and how much privacy will be afforded. The client is not only informed, but he also receives the message loudly and clearly that the nurse is sensitive to his needs, knows the technical aspects and expectations of the procedures, and considers him a person. The equipment should be assembled outside the immediate environment, if possible, particularly when discomfort is associated with the technical action, the requisite equipment is not prepackaged, considerable time is needed to prepare the equipment, or the nurse needs to take more time to organize and familiarize herself with the use of the equipment and the procedural method, or needs to consult someone about the technical aspects of its use or procedural method. If the technical aspects are to be performed by or in cooperation with another member of the health team, a mutual understanding of the role of each person (nurse, health professional, client) and the requisites for the procedure should be established in advance. The client's preparation and participation should be clarified before the technical action is initiated.

The nurse continually uses decision-making skills, judging when the procedural method and the timing of the technical action must be modified, or consultation with or assistance from other persons is necessary to assure a safe, effective action.

In each contact with the client, the nurse not only focuses on the purpose or goal of the interaction but also continually expands her perceptual ability to obtain data about the client indicating that the planned action is correct. She seeks data that would indicate other problems arising from unmet or poorly met basic human needs. She continually reviews the client's reaction to her thoughts and actions, for he quickly picks up discrepancies between verbal expressions of interest and concern and actual practice. When the client is not called by his name, or when the nurse fails to look at him, uses a brusque manner, is impatient, rough, or focuses on a body part or piece of equipment rather than on him, her disinterest in him as a person is clearly evident.

If another member of the nursing team assists the nurse with planned actions, special attention must be paid to the client-centered focus. Conversation between or among nursing personnel in the presence of the client should focus on and include him. Social conversation or conversation pertaining to other clients, or about nursing and health care personnel, has no place in the immediate client setting. Further, the client quickly picks up the nurse's and her assistant's lack of interest, attention, and concern. The impact may be quite serious if the client's ability to cope with the situation is strained, his concept of himself is low, and if he is apt to misinterpret motives. While light conversation may be very appropriate and may serve as needed diversion, it should include the client and be of interest to him.

> Lois Lawst, a 10-year-old girl with diabetes, was in the treatment room waiting for the nurse who was to teach her how to administer insulin. Two other nurses and two nursing students had accompanied the client to the treatment room after requesting her permission to observe her progress. During the waiting period, some questions were directed toward the young girl and, initially, the conversation included her. Shortly, however, the conversation drifted away from the client, and the four nurses soon became deeply involved in a personal conversation that portrayed a socioeconomic status far different from that of the 10-year-old. She sat alone and was temporarily forgotten. Only when the expected nurse arrived was attention directed back to the client. Lois refused to give herself insulin that day.

As the nurse proceeds to implement the nursing care plan, she learns more about the person, his reactions, his feelings, his strengths, his limitations, his coping ability, his preferences, his satisfactions, and his dissatisfactions. She learns his response to planned nurse actions, additional ways available to him and to the nurse to perform actions, the need for additional actions, and any untoward response to the planned actions. These data are synthesized and utilized to further develop the nursing care plan and are the basis for recording data about the client on appropriate nursing records.

If the nurse finds that some or selected actions should and could be performed safely by other members of the nursing team, she should delegate these actions. She knows the capabilities of nursing team members, and should also know the responsibilities of persons with a particular title as well as those who have a specific role. She needs to know the strengths and limitations of the individuals in these roles. She should focus on selecting the most appropriate person to perform a specific action for the client. The person so designated should have as much information about the client as she needs so that her actions are truly effective and the nursing team member is able to perform in an informed manner. Thus, delegated activities are part of the whole focus of action and contribute purposefully to immediate, intermediate, and long-range goals of care. The person performing the delegated tasks is responsible for her own acts and is expected to report the outcome in terms of the client. The nurse supervises the performance of supportive nursing personnel.[38-42] Data about the client obtained by team members should be communicated to the nurse responsible for his care and for implementing the nursing care plan. If more than one nurse is involved in the client's care, particularly in inpatient settings, written and verbal reports concerning the client as well as an up-to-date nursing care plan are needed to insure continuity and goal-direction. If each nurse is responsible for the client's care, each should participate in changes needed to keep the nursing care plan viable. If conflict arises relative to the interpretation of goals specific to the action to be taken by the nurse, the priority of action to meet the desired goal, or client responses differing at different times of the day, a conference should be planned with the nurses involved and with the client to resolve it. This does not necessarily mean that two different means could not be used to achieve the same end because the views, knowledge, or experiences of the nurses involved differed. Resolution is needed only when conflict involves a goal or priority opposing that planned with the client.

In designating the *who* in terms of planned nurse action, the nurse may feel that she is the best person to perform the action at a particular time. She may require assistance and will decide on who, the amount, and type of assistance she needs. She may delegate selected nurse actions to other nursing personnel. This pattern may vary from time to time, from day to day, and even from moment to moment—always dictated by behavioral changes in the client, available nurse manpower, and the coping ability of the client and his family.

The nurse gives care if she is the best prepared person to implement the particular action from an intellectual, interpersonal, and/or technical standpoint. She may find that her performance of a particular action will serve as a vehicle or means to meet needs for safety, love, and esteem. She may wish to use her presence—her thereness—to give the client an opportunity to express himself and to share his doubts, fears, and anxieties.

Just as the nurse's philosophy, education, and experience influenced the type and character of nursing actions she designed to meet problems, so will these significantly affect implementing the actions. Her emphasis, her focus, and her creativity will be affected by her own strengths, limitations, prejudices, stereotypes, her knowledge of human behavior, the strength of her convictions, her ability to handle human closeness, and her ability to use herself therapeutically. Her willingness to share her knowledge and give of herself, as well as her knowledge of her intellectual, emotional, social, and spiritual boundaries, will influence what the nurse will do, can do, and knows enough not to do.

Gentleness, sureness, and strength can be conveyed by the nurse, not only to alleviate associated discomfort, embarrassment, or frustration accompanying the problem, but to actually meet some basic human needs—love and safety.

If other persons are involved in the client's care, the nursing care plan gives direction to the actions of nursing and health care personnel. But the actions and activities of these persons need to be coordinated to make them person-centered and to make certain that vertical planning is implemented. Coordination takes into account who is doing what and when. This assures that actions are taken and that the client's biologic rhythms and his situation are benefited rather than overwhelmed. It is possible that an action may be ineffective simply because it is poorly timed, or is done in conjunction with other actions that may conflict or interfere with each other. For example, a health professional enters the room to treat a client with a poor appetite just as he begins to eat. Or she plans a care activity just as a visitor enters the room of a lonely client. Persons involved in activities with a client may influence the performance of a specific action because of the variation in approach. For example, the manner in which a client is helped out of bed, how he is supported, which side of the bed is used to get him out of it, and whether he is allowed to dangle before he gets up may influence his desire to get out of bed, the amount of time he spends out of bed, and what he does when he is out of bed.

Depending on the client's response during implementation, priorities may have to be reassigned, and reassessing and replanning will then be required. Nursing judgment is needed to know what to do with data, the additional data needed, what the data mean, whether a new nursing diagnosis is needed, and what the plan of action should be.

Thus, the implementation phase, although it does have an action focus, also includes assessing, planning, and evaluating activities by the nurse. The actions of implementation performed with and for the client could include the following: inserting, withdrawing, turning, cleansing, rubbing, massaging, flexing, irrigating, manipulating, teaching, exercising, offering, awakening, cuddling, holding, drying, applying, communicating, administering, influencing, altering, relieving, supporting, cooling, warming, providing, accompanying, sitting with, listening, walking, moving, touching, soothing, pulling, pushing, facilitating, interacting with, straightening, twisting, wrapping, folding, flexing, to mention a few. Strategic to these actions are those related to assessing, planning, and evaluating, which complement the action implemented. These actions are needed to resolve, diminish, or dissolve the client's problem.

The actions may be independent or interdependent functions of the nurse. The latter relate to carrying out doctor's orders for drugs and treatment, which are part of the medical care plan and collaborating with multidisciplinary health team members to effect a specific outcome. Interdependent functioning does not imply following orders of other health team members blindly and without question. Critical thinking and sound judgment must be exercised to make decisions about what, when, how much, and in what manner. For example, specific nurse action planned to relieve pain should follow a careful assessment of physiologic manifestations of the pain, its location, quality, and character, severity, what the pain being experienced means to the client, and other factors. The nurse needs to know the pattern of the pain, verbal and nonverbal evidences, and gestures. The nurse may be able to utilize pharmacologic measures and/or manipulate the client by changing his position, removing wrinkles or restrictions, and by taking actions that influence his behavioral response to pain. McCaffery summarized the physiologic and physical factors influencing the client's sensation of pain and his behavior associated with it as: (a) neurophysiologic processes underlying the sensation of pain, duration and intensity of pain, alterations in the level of consciousness, cutaneous versus visceral sites of pain, environmental conditions, sensory restriction, physical strain and fatigue; (b) cultural aspects, including sociocultural group membership, age, sex, religion, body part involved in the pain, roles ascribed to members of the health team; and (c) psychologic factors, including emotionally traumatic life experiences, secondary gains of the client's complaint of pain, personal past experience with pain, knowledge, understanding, and cognitive level, powerlessness, attitude and feeling of others, perceptual dominance of pain.[43] Thus, the client's pain involves more than automatically administering a prescribed analgesic when he states that he is in pain.

The implementation phase concludes when the nurse's actions are completed and she has recorded the results of actions and the client's reaction to them. Recording these actions and reactions is an important function of the nurse. The quality of the recording about the client and what the nurse chooses to document give direct evidence of the status of goal-achievement and individual client reactions, and designates the status of and the direction for continued problem-solving. Placing a low value on recording, or insufficient or inappropriate recording, is an affront to the client and demonstrates the nurse's limitations. Automatic notations or general statements give little or no indication of the client's individuality, his problem, and his reactions to the planned action. The recordings are related to the problem; they describe the nurse's actions and the results, and include additional data. The written report of nursing care given serves to direct continuing action. Communication—oral and written—associated with the nursing history and health assessment, nursing diagnosis, nursing orders or strategies and actions, client actions and reactions, should be given a high priority by the nurse. Her recording should reflect the client's unique situation and should be identified easily by the quality of their content. The recording should contain the information needed to give a profile of the client. Rules that set limits on what and how much should be recorded and that have only one basis—supposedly to save time—can be a waste of time. The nurse must decide what to write, how much to write, when to write, where to write, and that which is important. Where to write has the least significance compared with what and how much to write. The place is generally designated by the prevailing record system in an agency. If the prevailing record system is inadequate, action should be taken to institute a system worthy to receive the written observations and actions of the nurse. Writing associated with the development of the nursing history (including health assessment), nursing care plans, and recordings about an action performed is a professional, not a clerical, activity. Nor should it be delegated to persons who are not prepared to assume this important professional responsibility. Specific recording of data certainly may be delegated, but not the nursing history, the nursing care plan, or recording significant data about the client that stems from implementing the plan. Recordings are more frequent when the client's behavior changes rapidly. If these changes occur slowly and are infrequent, there will be less to record but the information will not lose its significance. When recordings become copious or their use is minimized because one does not have the time to review them, the information should be summarized periodically in coordination and in conjunction with the nursing care plan. It would be helpful to index recordings of client progress. The process of indexing would be based on significant experiences or stages in the resolution of a problem, and would also be useful for nursing care plans. If plans have been developed over long periods of time, a new or revised nursing care plan should be developed. All previous plans or additions to it should be retained as long as the client has problems that have not been resolved or that are being dealt with but cannot be resolved. Plans developed with persons who are well or for whom health prevention and maintenance are major goals will be reactivated, as needed, for reassessment. These plans and records should be retained for evaluative purposes and future planning.

Thus, the implementation phase of the nursing process includes nurse actions determined by the nursing care plan. The nurse continues to focus on the client, conveying, through her intellectual, interpersonal, and technical skills, that he is indeed worthy of her respect and is imbued with dignity. Nurse actions are based on scientific rationale and directed toward promoting a suitable internal and external environment in which wellness is enhanced and illness diminished. Factors in the external environment include influencing significant legislative actions, particularly those related to health and environment. Available resources and their appropriate use are inherent in the implementation phase. The appropriateness and direction of the nurse's action(s) are determined by the client's behavioral change in the direction of goal achievement. The direction and amount of change is evaluated.

Evaluating

Evaluation, the fourth component of the nursing process, follows the implementation of actions designated in the nursing care plan. Evaluation is *always considered in terms of how the client responded to the planned action.* Since specific nurse actions were planned to solve client problems, any judgment about how these problems are being resolved should originate with the client. It was noted earlier that the nursing diagnosis and the goal of resolution (expected outcome) of the client problem would serve as the framework for the evaluation component.

The nursing care plan contains the framework for evaluation. The impact of all intellectual, interpersonal, and technical actions on the client and the changes these produce are the focus of evaluation.

Although elements of evaluation, like those of assessment and planning, are concurrent and recurrent with other components, evaluating the effect of actions during and after the implementation phase determines the client's response and the extent to which immediate, intermediate, and long-range goals are achieved. The evaluation must continue in a purposeful, goal-directed manner. For example, if relief of pain is to be expected from implementing the nurse action, the results would be known within a short period of time. The client would tell the nurse that his pain was or was not relieved. The nurse could compare the client's behavior prior to nurse action, noting posture, facial expression, pulse and respiratory rates, color of a part, and his ability to focus on other topics and other persons rather than on the pain. There would be substantial behavioral evidence that would indicate that the client's pain was fully relieved and the nurse actions had brought about that relief; alternatively, the nurse could conclude that no pain relief or limited pain relief was obtained and her actions had been ineffective or only partially effective.

Evaluation is the natural intellectual activity completing the process phases because it indicates the degree to which the nursing diagnosis and nursing actions have been correct. By evaluating nursing actions the nurse demonstrates that she accepts responsibility for these actions and shows her interest and involvement in enhancing the effectiveness of actions directed toward solving the client's problems. It also demonstrates that the actions are person-centered and there is less likelihood a nurse action will be continued if it is not helpful.

Evaluation will also pinpoint omissions during the assessment, planning, and implementation phases. In any given client situation, it is possible that some problems may be resolved at different time intervals. Since evaluation will be in terms of immediate, intermediate, and long-range goals, the evaluation process is continued until these goals are realized. The outcome of the evaluation may indicate that the care planned must be reassessed, replanned, modified, and the revised plan implemented and evaluated. Thus, the nursing process is a continuing cycle.

The nurse and the client are the agents of evaluation. Other persons, such as the client's family, nursing personnel, and health team personnel, may also be involved. Based on the behavioral expectations of the client relative to the mutually agreed upon immediate, intermediate, and long-range goals, measurement data are collected so that value judgments can be made. A number of measuring devices and methods are available to obtain these data. These data include the following: temperature recording, pulse rate, blood pressure recording, apex rate, electrocardiogram and electroencephalogram recordings, and a gamut of physiologic analyses, such as urinalysis, blood sugar, blood urea nitrogen, and cholesterol. The condition and situation of the client–his posture, appearance, color, level of orientation and statements–made by his family and significant others knowledgable about his situation –should be used by the nurse in her evaluation. The nurse uses her senses to collect data; she utilizes communication techniques to elicit subjective data (questioning the client about dizziness and nausea), makes inferences and validates them, and makes a decision about the client's behavioral response.

The outcome of evaluation may be any one or a combination of the following:

1. The client responded as he had been expected to and his problem is resolved. No further nursing action is needed. A plan to maintain the client's state of optimal wellness is formulated jointly by the nurse and the client. An appointment may be made for a future date to reaffirm the client's problem-free status.
2. Behavioral manifestations of the client's situation indicate that his problem has not been resolved; evidence demonstrates that immediate goals but not intermediate and long-range goals have been achieved. The nature of the client's problem is such that complete resolution, if it is possible, will be slow. The nurse action is then geared to fulfillment of intermediate and long-range goals. These goals include preventing antic-

ipated and possible problems. Reevaluation will continue.

3. Behavioral manifestations of the client are similar to those evidenced during the assessment phase. Little or no evidence that his problem has been resolved is available. Immediate goals have not been realized; there may or may not be evidence that intermediate or long-range goals may begin to be realized. Anticipated and possible problems may or may not have been prevented. Reassessment with replanning is needed.
4. Behavioral manifestations indicate new problems. Assessment, planning, and implementing a plan of action to resolve this problem are in order. Planning action to resolve the new problem must be coordinated with the planning for the previously diagnosed problems. Evaluation will follow implementation.

If the nurse has used the logical, goal-directed problem-solving approach of the nursing process, evaluation should indicate a high level of success. Involving the client and his family in the nursing process contributes to this success. The likelihood that any or all of the client's problems will not be resolved is decreased.

As the nursing profession directs its efforts toward developing standards for the practice of nursing, these standards are broadly stated and are applicable to all clients who enter the health care system, particularly the nursing subsystem. Standards of nursing practice are stated in terms of a systematic, goal-directed, problem-solving approach. The profession fulfills its obligations to provide and improve nursing practice by developing these standards, which are now recognized by nurse practitioners. The standards convey to the citizenry a model of service that can be expected from members of the profession and their assistants. The nurse actions directed toward resolving client problems are guided by these standards, and action is measured and compared with the standards. Evaluation of nurse actions purposely directed toward the client's problem, as included in the nursing care plan, is applicable to a specific client.

As in all other phases, the client is involved in evaluation. Specific nurse actions may be found to be highly effective, moderately or minimally effective, or ineffective, but these conclusions can only be reached after the degree to which the client's problem has been resolved is evaluated, based on the behavioral manifestations he demonstrates. Judgment during other phases may have resulted in immediate reassessment and replanning. But only during the evaluation phase is a comprehensive appraisal of goal achievement —immediate, intermediate, long-range—made. After client behavior is evaluated, the quality of nursing care and its impact on the client's health status is determined.

Some of the questions the nurse can ask during this evaluation phase are: What was the expected client behavior? Was the expected behavior realistic, accurate? What data supported the judgment that the behavior was realistic and accurate? What behavior was manifested? What tools or instruments were utilized to obtain the data? What observable data were collected? What judgments were made concerning these data? Were significant data overlooked, omitted or devalued? What subjective data were collected and documented? Were data synthesized and compared before the value judgment was made? Does the client agree with the judgment? Do other members of the nursing team and health team concur with the value judgment?

What additional data are needed? How should they be obtained? From whom should they be obtained—the client, his family and associates, the nurse, doctor, clinical pharmacist, teacher, or employer? Are data needed from one or all of these sources?

Were the nursing diagnosis, nursing orders or strategies, and nursing care plans accurate and realistic? Was the plan of action accurate, but the action ineffective because it was not carried out accurately, was inept, or did not consider the client as a person? Was there input from the client? If not, why not? Was the nurse action accomplished by the wrong member of the nursing team? Was it a nurse action at all or should it have been accomplished by the client and/or his family members, or a member of the health team?

What goals—immediate, intermediate, long-range—have been or are being met? If goals have been met, what are the plans to periodically reassess and maintain a problem-free status?

What factors influenced goal attainment? What factors influenced the limited or lack of goal achievement? Were these factors internal and/or external to the client/his family, the nurse, nursing team members, health team members, other persons such as friends, neighbors, co-workers? What factors were related to the setting in which the nursing care took place—the home, the clinic, industry, a health care facility? Were environmental, socioeconomic, cultural, or religious factors involved?

Are some problems partially resolved? How is this partial response determined? Is it due to factors in the client's internal or external environment? Could the problem have been resolved completely if additional data have been sought or an alternative solution tried? Was the assessment complete? Was the nursing diagnosis correct? Did the problem resolve itself despite omissions in assessment, planning, and implementation? What contributed to this resolution?

If the client's behavioral manifestations indicate that his problem was not resolved, what were the reasons? Were there physiologic, psychologic, intellectual, socioeconomic, cultural, and religious reasons for the lack of resolution? What external factors are influencing this failure to solve his problem? Do the nursing care and medical care plans conflict rather than complement each other? Is there a lack of resources (human, financial, technical)? Is there a permanent handicap, an incomplete understanding of the problem and its impact?

Has the situation been labeled a problem when it is not a problem? Do the client and the nurse want to relinquish the problem? If nurse action was deemed appropriate but the results of the action were ineffective, what was the reason? Was timing incorrect? Did the appropriate member of the nursing team implement the action? Was consideration given to the age, sex, developmental level, and role of the client? Is the limitation in the nurse's intellectual, interpersonal, and/or technical skills or in those of a team member?

Was communication effective? Was the message received identical to that sent? Did feedback verify the accuracy of the message?

Did the client suffer an affront to his feelings as a person—failure to identify him by name, focusing on a part of rather than on the whole person, attending to equipment rather than the client, ignoring persons significant to the client and their participation in his care? Was recognition given to the psychologic, emotional, religious, cultural, and socioeconomic influences inherent in the client situation and accompanying implementation of nurse actions?

Was the intent of the goals clear—immediate, intermediate, and long-range? Are new problems evident? Are they related to other unresolved client problems? Are they unrelated? What data are available about the new problem? Is the problem known to the client? What is his reaction? Is the new problem the result of new pathology or changed socioeconomic status? Is it the result of nearsightedness in anticipating problems? Is it the result of a change in the client's role, his diminished ability to cope with his situation, or a change in body image? Are there changes within the family system?

Are there previous problems that have not been dealt with? How have long-range plans influenced these problems? Have they been realistic? Have these plans and related actions made an impact?

Were the immediate, intermediate, and long-range goals geared to preventing disease and maintaining health as well as to sickness care, if needed?

Were the nursing actions based on principles from the physical, biologic and behavioral sciences? Was the nurse action stifled by a rigid policy interpretation, failure to accept the fact that there are independent functions of the nurse?

When the data for evaluation are collected, analyzed, and synthesized a new picture emerges. The nursing care plan may continue as designed or it may need to be revised partially or completely. Additions may be made or alternative action selected. The client situation may indicate a transfer to a health care facility (from a general hospital to a nursing home or vice versa) or even a transfer to another unit of the same health care facility (from intensive care to a surgical unit).

Changes in the client situation or location within the health care system may involve other health professionals. The balance of action geared toward maintaining wellness, preventing illness, giving care during sickness, or fostering rehabilitation may show a directional shift toward the client or toward the nurse.

Once the new status (direction of change and progress toward goal achievement) is designated, based on the evaluation, either the problem is resolved and no further nurse action is needed or new priorities are set and goals determined. Modification is incorporated in the evaluation phase and follows it. Modification results in reprocessing activity, feeding back to assessment for reassessment, and continuing the cycle of each phase. The cyclic process is continued as long as it is needed; in other words, as long as there are goals to be achieved or until the client completes his life span. If the goal that is to be achieved is to maintain the client's well status, periodic reassessment may continue for an unlimited time span. The nurse-client relationship may reflect periodicity rather than a continuous hour-by-hour interaction.

In viewing the use of the nursing process with a client longitudinally, the time interval of nurse-client interactions may demonstrate periodic, continuous, or any combination of periodic and continuous interactions, as evidenced by the client's wellness-illness profile over a span of years.

The act of evaluating may be strengthened and clarified by the following examples. An interaction was heard one morning in the nurses' station of a coronary care unit. Three nurses had the following conversation:

> **Nurse A:** (leafing through the client's chart). I think we should talk about Mr. Klotz. He's the client with a myocardial infarction, who came in two nights ago. This morning it was the same thing again. Complaints and more complaints. He says he can't sleep with a light on; the night nurse is too noisy; he is awakened when he just about dozes off, and the aide always bumps his bed when she goes in to do something.
>
> **Nurse B:** What does Mr. Klotz expect in the coronary care unit? He is not the only one here. Last night there was a cardiac arrest, so naturally there would be a lot more excitement. He isn't even as sick as some of the other patients are. And the lights aren't bright. They are dimmed after 8:00. We could tell the aide not to be so clumsy. I think we should spend time talking about the sicker clients or taking care of clients.
> **Nurse C:** Mr. Klotz should give his complaints to the night nurse where they belong.
>
> **Nurse A:** (leafing through the client's chart) I disagree! Mr. Klotz may really be saying that he is very frightened of the night. Maybe he thinks he will die. And look at this! Did you notice that his pulse is higher at bedtime and during the early morning hours than it is during the day? This is documented by the monitor strip on the nurse's notes. His respirations are increased, too, and he is perspiring and pale. When I first see him in the morning he looks anxious. His anxiety seems to be having an affect on his cardiovascular system.
>
> **Nurse B:** That's interesting! I hadn't noticed this relationship. Maybe he is telling us something and we almost missed the message.
>
> **Nurse C:** Yes, maybe we should ask the night nurse to join our conference so we could pool our observations and plan an approach to verify if Mr. Klotz is anxious and why. Then maybe we could help him.

This example points up the use of specific measures to verify behavioral change.

In the following example, the nurse concluded that she had adequately taught an expectant mother to bathe an infant when she observed the woman do so effectively.

The nurse was present when 20-year-old Mrs. Noo bathed an infant during a prenatal class demonstration period. When the nurse observed the client bathing her own infant during a postnatal visit to her home, Mrs. Noo demonstrated the ability to follow through safely and effectively during the bath. She had assembled all necessary items, and handled the infant firmly, yet gently and lovingly. Mrs. Noo reported what she knew and what additional information she needed. The nurse had specific data on which to judge that a specific goal had been achieved. These data were specific behaviors demonstrated by Mrs. Noo, as observed by the nurse.

While on a home visit to assess the needs of a diabetic teenager, the nurse noted that the teenager's mother seemed worried and preoccupied. Validating her observation, the nurse found that Mrs. Frite, a 43-year-old widow and mother of three teenagers was most fearful of her own safety. She told the nurse that her mother had died of cancer of the cervix a year ago and her oldest sister was to have a hysterectomy for a cervical malignancy. Though Mrs. Frite expressed her fear of cancer, she refused any suggestion that she have a pelvic examination and a cytologic smear. If the expected behavior resulting from the nurse's action to relieve this fear of cancer was that Mrs. Frite would accept this advice, make an appointment with a gynecologist, and keep the appointment, it would have been specific behavioral evidence that the nurse's goals had been realized. The immediate goal was to give Mrs. Frite an opportunity to verbally express her fears of cancer and a cytologic smear, provide specific information about the smear, and assess the availability of a gynecologist in her area. Within two weeks, Mrs. Frite did follow the nurse's suggestion. Both examinations were negative for pathology, and Mrs. Frite was very relieved.

If the client has difficulty remaining oriented because of sensory deprivation, behavioral evidence within the client must be sought to demonstrate whether the deprivation was relieved. By comparing the client's behavioral profile before and after nursing action, needed data are obtained to make an evaluative judgment. The basis of sensory deprivation may be factors within the client. He may have a sensory deficit—unable to see, hear, or speak. He may be very young or very old; there may be pathophysiologic and psychopathologic reasons. He may be isolated from the mainstream of activity due to disease or therapy (staphylococcal infection, radiation treatment), or by geographic location. He may lack appeal; he may not look good, smell good, or have wholesome habits. He may have no relatives or friends; he may be unconscious, nonverbal, and withdrawn. If the problem were diagnosed and a series of nurse actions were planned to relieve the deprivation, evidence of increased orientation, cerebration, and sociability would be some of the behaviors the nurse would expect to see in the client. Of course, behavioral expectations would be those of which the client would be capable. Behavioral manifestations of lessened sensory deprivation for the unconscious client would need to be specified and observed.

If the client is expected to verbally express who he is, where he is, plan what he wants to do and then do it, or plan and know when and why he cannot follow through, the nurse will have a series of behaviors that designate a decrease in sensory deprivation and an increase in sensory input. (See Appendix D for sample of nursing process referring to sensory deprivation as the nursing diagnosis.) Expecting the client to demonstrate that he is oriented in a way in which he was not capable at any time previously would result in failure to achieve a goal. For example, if a child is disoriented, expecting him to tell time and know the date may be beyond that which he is able to accomplish, considering his age and level of growth and development.

Nurses have supplied calendars and clocks; these are particularly needed if the client is in a room that does not have a window. A radio is helpful since time checks, weather reports, news events, as well as a variety of voice tones or music may stimulate the client in whom sensory deprivation is a problem. These aids are especially useful for the unconscious or blind person, and serve as adjuncts to human interaction on the verbal and nonverbal level.

The nurse will seek evidence that the client can recognize familiar and significant persons and things. She can observe the number of human contacts the client has and the quality of the interaction. Does anyone speak to the client or touch him? Does he experience variations in sensation, such as coolness, warmth, softness, roughness, smoothness?

What are the sounds, smells, sights, colors, temperature of the environment? What are the furnishings of the environment? What sensory stimulation is there for the client? Is he an active or passive recipient of this stimulation? Does he attempt sensory stimulation himself?

Is the client lethargic, unresponsive, irritable, despairing? Does he complain about limited human contacts? Is there a clock or a calendar he can see, is there a radio or television set in his room and is one or the other turned on? If the client is unconscious, does the nurse talk to him and tell him what she does when she lifts his leg or his arm or elevates the bed? Does she tell him the water is cold, warm, or if compresses are placed on his body? Does she tell him the time of day, day of the week, month of the year? Does the client hear various voice tones—masculine, feminine, loud, soft? These might be some of the questions that must be answered to evaluate changes in client responses, using the initial assessment as a baseline. The results may indicate less sensory deprivation, indicating that the nursing actions planned should be continued. Modification in terms of the kind of nursing action, the person doing the action, the intensity and timing of action, increasing the length of human contact, changing the quality of the contact, and increasing the number of persons involved, may be necessary.

If the client is a child and excessive crying was diagnosed as a lack of need fulfillment, then crying should decrease after nurse actions planned to fulfill physiologic, safety, and love needs have been implemented. The actual amount of time spent in crying, the character of the cry, the amount of playful activity, evidence of contentment, improved appetite, and increased weight would be observed, recorded, and used to judge that the child's needs were being fulfilled. Nurse actions would be considered appropriate, based on the behavioral change noted in the client.

It is expected that if the nursing process is the key to solving these problems affecting the client's wellness or illness, its use should be highly effective. Supporting the degree to which success was expected is the fact that the nursing process is systematic, logical, and goal-directed, focusing on the client and his situation. The client is considered the nurse's partner throughout the phases of the process. In instances where goals have not been fully achieved and when a judgment has been made that a particular nurse action or series of nurse actions had little or no effect on the problem for which it was planned, as demonstrated by client behavior, the nurse looks for the reason.

Sources for reasons why predicted outcomes were not realized include the client, the nurse, significant others (to the client), nursing staff members, and health team members.

Concerning the client, possible causes include sharing inaccuracies, insufficient information, or withholding important data about self and situation. Causes for failures to realize goals can include an increase in pathophysiology and/or psychopathology, allergic manifestations, a drain on the client's expected ability to cope with his problem due to multiple influencing variables acting simultaneously. Unrealistic expectations of one's self and predicament, loss of self-esteem, loss of job, inadequate finances, untoward reaction to therapeutic agents—chemical, mechanical, pharmacologic—a lack of or an insufficient opportunity to participate in diagnosing problems and planning strategies, failure to seek immediate attention for high priority problems, a lack of interest in and attention to intermediate and long-range goals, and planned strategies and goals that have not been accepted are other reasons.

If the nurse is the source, the reasons why the client's problem has not been resolved may include overlooking data; assigning high or low priorities inappropriately; a failure to validate a hunch or inference; a lack of knowledge about the client's situation, particularly socioeconomic, cultural, and religious; failure to recognize intellectual, interpersonal, and technical limitations; failure to use intellectual, interpersonal, and technical strengths; inappropriate delegation of nurse actions to nursing team members; failure to consider elements of the medical plan when formulating the nursing care plan; limited sharing of important information about the client with health team members; failure to consider the value of input from family members, employers, or teachers; excessive focus on dependent functions; inadequate fulfillment of independent and interdependent nursing functions; deficiencies in taking a nursing history and performing a health assessment; failure to involve the client in planning; failure to recognize client strengths and his need for independence within the limits of his wellness or illness; ineffective and/or infrequent communication; failure to consider significant others; and failure to recognize the impact the nurse makes on others.

For nursing team members, possible reasons contributing to ineffective goal achievement may be insufficient information about the client and his problem, his expectations, or his goals; failure to convey important data about the client to the nurse who is responsible for the care plan; interpersonal affronts to the client as a person—not calling him by name, failure to insure his privacy and that of his messages, conversing in his presence without including him; failure to record important data such as intake-output or changes in quality and rate of pulse; giving information about the client to a nurse not knowledgeable about the client; focusing on things rather than on the client; being noisy, loud, insensitive, and forceful or domineering.

Concerning the significant others of the client, some of the reasons goals are not achieved are: they are not available or are not interested in the client; his problem, the solution, and expected behavioral change are not understood; the client has a limited ability to cope with his problem; fears and anxieties exist about self and client; they fail to see that a problem exists or resources

–financial, physical and emotional energy, intellectual endowment –are limited; lack of transportation; and moral, cultural, and religious influences.

Health team members may be responsible for the failure to achieve the goals planned for the client. Reasons for failures in these cases might include a conflict of goals for the client, failure to discern when the focus is upon a part of the client rather than the whole, inability to function as a team member, failure to see value in a nursing care plan, limited experience in communicating with members of the nursing team and other health team members, focus on technical aspects of contribution to the exclusion of the interpersonal component, and acts of depersonalizing the client.

Other facets of evaluation have been developed in recent years and continue to merit attention. Presently, considerable pressure is being exerted by the recipients of health and nursing care for accountability with regard to services rendered. The nursing process is just such a vehicle to demonstrate accountability that the care rendered is appropriate to the client's total health care needs, that it is moral, economical, and that the desired results have been achieved, i.e., need fulfillment to an optimal level for the client.

A formal and systematic program developed and implemented to determine quality client care is termed *health care quality assurance*. A total quality assuarnce program should provide for input from the client, his family, the nurse and her peers, and other health care workers. Efforts have been exerted by nurses and other health personnel involved in rendering health services to clients to determine the level of quality of health and nursing services and to establish whether these services make a difference in outcome for the client. The nurse peer review is one method whereby practicing nurses, as peers, appraise the quality of client care rendered by equally qualified practitioners of nursing. This review (focusing on the developed nursing process and client behavioral outcomes) is based on prestated criteria or standards, thereby determining the level of quality of care. This review may be geared to one peer or to a group of peers in a specific health care agency. Such a review should benefit all clients as well as specific clients and should provide a means of evaluation over and above the ongoing evaluation of the nurse's ability to assess, plan, implement, and evaluate nursing care by one's superiors. The expected outcomes for the nurse peer review are (1) the support of a high level of client care; (2) the diagnosis of low level care with definitive plans developed for implementation to offset the deficiency; (3) the accumulation of precise data to justify employment of prepared nurses capable of expert utilization of the nursing process and in a number sufficient to meet the health and nursing goals for clients; (4) direct feedback to individual nurses about care rendered by them; and (5) data to support and designate areas of need for orientation programs, inservice education, and continuing education.

A number of tools have been developed and tested for use in concurrent and retrospective evaluation of client care. These tools may be applied to the total client population or to a random sample. These samples should be selected on the basis of nursing diagnoses. Nurse peer review should follow an established pattern that is continuous rather than one that occurs once a year or at unstructured intervals.

R. C. Jelinek et al. developed a most useful methodology for monitoring quality of nursing care based on the *nursing process* and *client needs* while simultaneously considering the persons, activities, and environmental elements that impinge on direct care as well as the administrative and organizational structure for the delivery of care.[44] This validated and reliable methodology utilizes the computer to generate work sheets and analyze data and allows for comparative interpretation of quality indices across health care agencies. Intensive testing and analyzing of the quality instrument has demonstrated it to be valid and reliable. The results of testing have demonstrated that the nursing process relates to client outcomes, and that identified variables such as registered nurse hours per client day, continuity of care, and coordination of parts of the patient care system related positively to quality care, whereas size and patient census per unit and nonprofessional staffing related negatively to quality care.[45]

Another instrument in use is the Quality Patient Care Scale (Qualpacs) developed by Wandelt and Ager to evaluate quality of nursing care received by clients while the care is in progress. In addition to measuring objectively the quality of interactions and interventions of nurses, it can be used to measure effects of changes in care, compare quality of care when differing staffing patterns are used, appraise the effects of inservice education, and provide data for research purposes as well as point up researchable problems.[46]

A tool for evaluation, developed, refined, and increasingly utilized by nurses, is the *nursing audit. Audit* usually suggests periodic inspection or review of records or accounts to insure honesty and accuracy in business transactions over a particular period of time. *Nursing audit* suggests, too, an inspection or review of some type of transaction. Potential areas of nursing that can be audited are assessment data and nursing diagnoses, nursing care plans, resulting client care, and a retrospective type in which the client's legal record of care is audited. A nursing audit is a review, by a nurse, of the client's care or his records to determine the extent to which that care and/or records meet established standards.

Auditing care plans developed for a client assume that the client's status has been assessed, a nursing history and health assessment have been done, a nursing diagnosis(es) has been made, the expected outcomes have been established, and nursing orders or strategies have been written to assure realization of the desired outcome. The recorded nursing care plans can be audited periodically by nurses who are less familiar with the client. The advantage of this type of audit is that it is probably an objective means for determining gaps in the plan or raising questions about areas of care that should be pursued, or areas of the plan that can be approached in another way.

The client's care can be audited by observing him when that care has been completed. A semicomatose person in a hospital can be observed for such aspects of care as body position, body cleanliness, status of the environment, apparent comfort. An ambulatory amputee in a clinic can be observed to detect the correct use of body mechanics, the care given to the body area near the prosthesis, and exercising techniques. A diabetic can be observed in his own home as he administers insulin to himself to determine how well he understands the instruction given him about insulin administration.

Records tell the auditor that data have been documented; to be certain of the quality of care that has been given, the most economic, effective, and direct way to audit this information is to observe the client. This offsets the question of whether the nurse who keeps detailed, well-written records also provides good nursing care. Auditing the care given to him is a certain and sure way to determine the extent to which that care has met established standards. The results of the audit can have direct implications for the client under care here and now.

Following the care of any client, some type of documentation is done on a legal record; the specific type of record depends on the setting in which the care is provided. A review of these legal records is the nursing audit performed most frequently. It is a client-centered activity and is a form of hindsight or retrospective evaluation. Phaneuf[47] developed the nursing audit process which is applicable to a variety of settings, and which has as its theoretical framework the independent and dependent functions of nursing. She developed this process to determine the extent to which nursing care has measured up to the specified objectives; it is not designed to evaluate care while it is being given, nor is it designed to be used to evaluate the nurse's performance.[47]

The persons responsible for the nursing audit are the professional nurses who can function as individual auditors or as a group of auditors. They may be associated closely with the client, be completely unfamiliar with the client, or the group may be composed of some nurses who know and some who do not know the client. The first task of the auditors is to establish standards against which their observations will be measured. While several nurses may be responsible for developing these standards, performing the audit or aspects of it can be delegated to various members of the group. It is important that peers review the final audit data and draw conclusions with determination of the required follow-up on the data.

The frequency with which audits are taken can be determined by the group, according to the type of client whose care is to be audited. The records of a critically ill person in a hospital will have to be audited more frequently than those of a person in a clinic. The care of chronically ill persons in a nursing home can be audited more regularly and less frequently than that of clients in a facility designed for the acutely ill. Important factors in the conduct of the audit are that nurses should be convinced of its value, should develop standards and auditing instruments appropriate to clients for whom they are responsible, and should be motivated to continue to improve the auditing techniques for their own satisfaction and especially for the continued improvement of the care given to the client.

The audit contributes to a systematic method for evaluating client care and assigning a qualitative judgment to the care and services received by a client. The nursing audit serves to pursue excellence and to contribute to the nurse's moral and legal accountability for the service she renders.

The nursing audit can not only contribute to an improved quality of nursing care, but can also influence the total health care system. It can contribute to better communication among and collaboration with nursing and health team members. The results of the audit should be shared with all persons concerned with client care. This openness, coupled with a knowledge of the goals of the auditing process, is strategic if the nursing care rendered is to be enhanced continuously and the quality of person-centered health care increased. It may provide data needed to effect required changes in the health care system.

Thus, the fourth component of the nursing process, evaluation, for which the framework has been prescribed, stems from the nursing care plan. Evaluation is always expressed in terms of achieving expected behavioral manifestations within the client. The entire focus of the nursing process is goal-directed. It is systematically geared to solve diagnosed client problems by prescribing specific nurse actions which would most successfully induce a specific behavioral effect that would denote the client's problem had been resolved.

Evaluation aids the nurse and client to determine problems that have been resolved, those that need to be reprocessed (which includes reassessment and replanning), and the diagnosis of new problems.

The need for research and for testing solutions to client problems is heavily supported through the use of the nursing process. Data about the client, gleaned through the process, can be used in nursing research.

References

1. Barrett-Lennard GT: Significant aspects of helping relationships. Mental Health (Canada) Special Suppl 47:1–5, 1965
2. Maslow A: Motivation and Personality. New York, Harper & Row, 1970
3. Montagu A: The Direction of Human Development, New York, Hawthorn, 1970
4. Erikson EH: Childhood and Society. New York, Norton, 1963, pp 247–274
5. Black K: Assessing patient needs. In Yura H, Walsh M: The Nursing Process, 1st ed., Washington, DC, The Catholic University of America Press, 1967, pp 1–20
6. Barrett-Lennard,[1] p 3
7. Frankl V: Man's Search for Meaning. New York, Washington Square Press, 1963
8. Erikson,[4] pp 247–274
9. Paterson J, Zderad L: Humanistic Nursing. New York, Wiley, 1976, p 4
10. Brown M, Fowler G: Psychodynamic Nursing. Philadelphia, Saunders, 1971, pp 21–23
11. Barrett-Lennard,[1] pp 1–2
12. *Ibid,* pp 3–4
13. Family Coping Index, Developed by Johns Hopkins School of Hygiene and Public Health and Richmond Instructive Visiting Nurse Asso-

ciation—City Health Department, Nursing Service (Richmond-Hopkins Cooperative Nursing Study), Directed by Freeman RB, 1964
14. Levine M: Adaptation and assessment: a rationale for nursing intervention. Am J Nurs 66:2450–2453, November 1966
15. Brown E: Newer Dimensions of Patient Care: Patients as People, Part 3. New York, Russell Sage Foundation, 1964
16. Maslow,[2]
17. Montagu A: On Being Human. New York, Hawthorn, 1966, pp. 49–52
18. Erikson,[4]
19. Duvall EM: Family Development. Philadelphia, Lippincott, 1971
20. Mayers M: A Systematic Approach to the Nursing Care Plan. New York, Appleton-Century-Crofts, 1972
21. Smith DM: A clinical nursing tool. Am J Nurs 68:2384–2388, November 1968
22. Lewis L: Planning Patient Care. Dubuque, Iowa, Brown, 1970, pp 35–62, 57–62
23. Little D, Carnevali D: Nursing Care Planning, 2nd edition. Philadelphia, Lippincott, 1976
24. Samuels M, Bennett H: The Well Body Book. New York, Random House, 1973
25. Chambers W: Nursing diagnosis. Am J Nurs 62:102–104, November 1962
26. Durand M, Prince R: Nursing diagnosis: process and decision. Nurs Forum 5(4):50–64, 1966
27. Gebbie K, Lavin MA: Classification of Nursing Diagnoses. St. Louis, Mosby, 1975
28. Gordon M: Nursing diagnoses and the diagnostic process. Am J Nurs 76:1298–1300, August 1976
29. Smith DM: Writing objectives as a nursing practice skill. Am J Nurs 71:319–320, February 1971
30. National League for Nursing. Problem-oriented Systems of Patient Care. New York, National League for Nursing, 1974
31. Mayers,[20]
32. Smith,[29]
33. Lewis,[22]
34. Johnson M, Davis M, Bilitch M: Problem-solving in Nursing Practice. Dubuque, Iowa, Brown, 1970
35. National League for Nursing [30]
36. Luce GG: Body Time. New York, Bantam, 1971
37. Harmer B: Methods and Principles of Teaching the Principles and Practice of Nursing. New York, Macmillan, 1926
38. Kron T: The Management of Patient Care. Philadelphia, Saunders, 1971
39. Douglass L, Bevis EO: Team Leadership in Action. St. Louis, Mosby, 1974
40. Lambertsen EC: Nursing definition and philosophy precede nursing goal development. Mod Hosp 103–136, 1964

41. Yura H, Ozimek D, Walsh M: Nursing Leadership: Theory and Process. New York, Appleton-Century-Crofts, 1976
42. Yura H, Walsh M: Super-vision. Superv Nurse 2:18–36, March 1971
43. McCaffery M: Nursing Management of the Patient with Pain. Philadelphia, Lippincott, 1972, pp 27–65
44. Jelinek RC, Haussman RKD, Hegyvary ST, Newman JF: A Methodology for Monitoring Quality of Nursing Care. Bethesda, Maryland, US Department of Health, Education and Welfare. Public Health Service. Health Resources Administration, Bureau of Health Resources Development, Division of Nursing, 1974, p 23
45. Haussman RKD, Hegyvary ST, Newman JF: Monitoring Quality of Nursing Care. Bethesda, Maryland, US Department of Health, Education, and Welfare, Public Health Service. Health Resources Administration, Bureau of Health Manpower, Division of Nursing, 1976, p 64
46. Wandelt M, Ager J. Quality Patient Care Scale. New York. Appleton-Century-Crofts, 1976, p 33
47. Phaneuf M: The Nursing Audit. Self-Regulation in Nursing Practice. New York, Appleton-Century-Crofts, 1976

Chapter Four •

Application of the Nursing Process

The nursing process can be applied in a variety of settings; it is flexible and adaptable, permitting the nurse to use judgment and creativity in caring for the client in an organized, orderly, and systematic manner.

A number of situations are presented in this chapter to illustrate (a) the variety of clinical and environmental settings in which the nursing process can be utilized, and (b) the variety of ways in which the nursing process can be used. Several situations have been selected for presentation. A few show how the nursing process was used after initial attempts failed to achieve the goals set for the client. One situation is presented in the first person—the nurse involved in caring for a terminally ill person reports her experience. One situation presents the client's thoughts about himself and then the nurse's thoughts about the client's problems, each in the first person. Other situations are presented in the third person—these are reports of how the nursing process was used to resolve the client's problems.

There is no stereotyped "one-way-only" to proceed through the phases of the process; nor is there a definite pattern to follow in moving back and forth among and between the different phases. These are factors that are determined according to the needs of the client in each situation, and the abilities of the individual nurse. Some situations deal with several facets of client care, others deal with a limited number of problem areas.

The never-ending challenge of coping with the many parameters of human behavior constantly stimulates and motivates nurses to improve their methods of client care. Some comments appear after the facts about each situation are presented. These are only a few of the possible comments that can be made. The reader, especially the learner, is encouraged to provide additional dimensions to the recorded comments.

• *Situation: Mrs. Ross in a Military Hospital* *

I said "Hello" to Mrs. Ross over a new, hand-breathing machine and she showed me how it was used. We said "Goodbye" three months later. Some of the things that occurred between the "Hello" and "Goodbye" I want to share with you. Particular emphasis will be focused on her pain and the consequences of pain.

"How well she explained the use of the machine," I thought. With several more inhalations and exhalations she completed her task. She leaned back in bed, savoring the momentary comfort it provided. Looking at me with warm brown eyes she asked, "Why haven't you been around before? I like your smile. It makes me feel good." Without waiting for a reply, her eyes sought those of the head nurse and said, "Captain Thomas makes over me and spoils me—I love it." Captain Thomas laughed and said, "You're easy to spoil." We continued to chat for a few more minutes and then I left her room. I did not realize then that this was the first of many times I'd be seeing and working with this lady.

When we returned to the nursing station, Captain Thomas, the head nurse, told me more about Mrs. Ross, a widow of some fifteen years. Her work in public services, until she became ill, was performed in Europe. She knew her job, every facet of it. Her illness began approximately nine months ago, when she developed constant right flank pain and intermittent gross hematuria. At that time, excretory urograms, cystograms, and cystoscopy were within normal limits. Because of her per-

* From LTC Madelaine Bader, ANC. Journal of Thanatology, Vol. II, No. 2, 1973. Courtesy of the author and Health Sciences Publishing Corporation.

sistent symptoms, subsequent excretory urograms were performed which showed progressive decreased function on the right side, with normal cystoscopy examination and normal bilateral retrograde ureterograms. Finally, because symptoms continued to persist, all tests were again repeated. An associated progressive problem of hypertension, requiring medication of hydrodiuril and reserpine, evidenced intermittent exacerbations. Mrs. Ross was transferred from Europe to the United States in December for further evaluation. Captain Thomas told me that Mrs. Ross intended to return to work as soon as possible. Illness, said she, was her enemy and she did not tolerate ill health with any degree of equanimity. She was a strikingly handsome woman, with lovely white hair that was ever so slightly waved. Her attitude was regal, yet warm and responsive. Although sixty-one she appeared to be in her early fifties. In December, she weighed 133 pounds. When I met her in March, she had lost twenty-five pounds. She carried her 5′6″ height gracefully. Every movement was executed with poise that completely lacked artificiality—even when she became quite ill, this quality never left her.

I must back up a bit and let you know how I first became involved with Mrs. Ross. Every fourth or fifth weekend, I, as well as other clinical chiefs, represent the Chief Nurse in her absence. One of our duties is to make rounds throughout the hospital. It was while making rounds on the urology unit that I met Mrs. Ross.

Previous to our actual meeting, I had heard Mrs. Ross' name mentioned quite often during morning report in the chief nurses' office. Since admission to Walter Reed General Hospital, she had undergone surgery for removal of her right kidney. During surgery, Mrs. Ross had a cardiac arrest, was resuscitated, and surgery was completed. The pathology report subsequently revealed adenocarcinoma with involvement of the right adrenal and vena cava. Two days after surgery, Mrs. Ross' vital signs were stable. The major problem, at that time, seemed to indicate possible renal failure. Several days later, hourly urine output had decreased markedly and Mrs. Ross was transferred from the intensive care unit to the renal unit. She required dialysis therapy for the next three days until urinary output could again be maintained by the patient. During her stay on the renal unit, morning reports indicated that Mrs. Ross was often observed crying or making cryptic comments about the patient with whom she shared the room. She wanted the patient moved to another area as she felt she needed to be alone to get the rest she required. Consistent remarks made in morning report were how "anxious" this lady appeared and how nursing staff was becoming increasingly more perplexed and frustrated over her apparent "unreasonable" demands or responses to any information or requests made of her.

My thoughts, after hearing repeated reports of Mrs. Ross' behavior and the vivid descriptions rendered by nurses reporting her condition, conjured forth a mental image of the usual stereotype—a rather cantankerous, fault-finding, demanding lady whose life style probably was in keeping with her present behavior and who no doubt was the proud possessor of three heads—all monsters.

I could scarcely believe that the Mrs. Ross I had met could be the same Mrs. Ross. I felt compelled to check with the head nurse to discover if the person was indeed she. Captain Thomas confirmed my query. "Yes, it's the same Mrs. Ross. She was transferred back to us yesterday. She's really happy to be back. I think when she saw patients receiving dialysis treatment she may well have had visions that her remaining life might consist of the same kinds of therapy." (Some days later this assumption was confirmed by Mrs. Ross as she shared, with me, some of the stresses patients could do without.)

Several busy weeks passed and I only vaguely wondered how Mrs. Ross was doing. One Monday morning I heard Captain Thomas' voice over the phone saying, "Hi, Colonel Bader, I think we could use some help with Mrs. Ross. I understand you are one of the founders of a project that's designed to help us work more effectively with terminally ill patients and with their families." * "That's right, Captain Thomas. You mentioned Mrs. Ross. . . ." "Yes, the doctors feel her prognosis is grave. Metastasis has begun and her condition is such that they feel the only care that can now be given will be of a supportive type."

When I asked for more information about Mrs. Ross, Captain Thomas poured out a multitude of facts and feelings. Mrs. Ross' daughters were here. The doctors had informed them of their mother's condition and prognosis. She felt both daughters accepted the news, but Sandy, the married daughter who had just arrived from Texas, appeared to be angry and unable to release any of her anger. Kitty, the single daughter who had

* PROJECT CAM (Crisis Awareness and Management) a project founded by a nurse and social worker to meet needs of terminally ill patients and their families as well as others who may be in crisis from lesser manifestations of loss, i.e., limb, organ, role, or relationship. Teaching seminars are conducted with interdisciplinary participants, designed to assist them in dealing with their own feelings about death and to increase their awareness and sensitivity so they would become more effective in meeting the needs of terminally ill patients and their families. On requests from units, we go to the unit and assist staff members in problem-solving. Guidelines and approaches are suggested, which they might utilize in meeting the needs of the patient and his family.

been with her mother off and on since admission, appeared concerned with the ways she could help her mother during this critical period. I learned from Captain Thomas that she had told the daughters about me and they expressed a desire to meet me. I arranged with Captain Thomas to meet with the daughters the following day. We scheduled a meeting with staff members for Thursday. Captain Thomas indicated that Dr. Lyons, the resident working with Mrs. Ross, planned to attend the meeting.

Thursday I was on the unit a few minutes early. Captain Thomas introduced me to Dr. Lyons, while other members of the staff brought chairs into the combination doctor-secretary office which would serve as our conference room. I met the other staff members, and added to the introduction Captain Thomas gave me by briefly explaining how the meeting came about and what I knew thus far about Mrs. Ross. I asked the staff members how I might be of assistance to them. They indicated their concern that Mrs. Ross, to the best of their knowledge, had not been informed of the seriousness of her condition. They felt they were in a bind, not knowing what to say or to do for Mrs. Ross. Their anger was directed towards Dr. Doe who had complete charge of her case. Dr. Lyons commented that Dr. Doe could not bring himself to tell Mrs. Ross about her prognosis, even when she asked. He and Dr. Doe had discussed "leveling" with her many times. Dr. Lyons felt Dr. Doe should tell her about her condition when she asks, without taking all her hope away. Dr. Doe apparently vacillates between telling her or keeping it from her, using as an argument that he really wasn't quite convinced the cancer had metastases —besides she never "really" asked him what was wrong with her. Staff members remarked that Dr. Doe has recently been seeing Mrs. Ross less frequently and stays only a short time. When he visits he seemed always accompanied by other doctors, and they wondered if this indicated his reluctance to be alone with her, for fear of the questions she might ask him. Staff members wanted to know how they should respond to Mrs. Ross if she asked them, "Am I going to die?" I wondered aloud if she had asked any of them that question. Captain Thomas was the only one that replied affirmatively. "She asked me. This was the other day when she was so wretched after repeated episodes of nausea and vomiting." She said, "Things look serious don't they?" "She waited for my answer and I just looked at her, nodded my head and touched her hand. She sort of sighed quietly and requested to see the legal officer. She wanted to make a statement donating her body, in case of death, to Walter Reed General Hospital."

We discussed how staff members might react if Mrs. Ross had posed this question to them. Some staff members indicated they would not be able to deal with such an inquiry, and besides, "she has never given me the slightest hint she thought she was going to die."

The need to deny operates within personnel as well as within the patient. If the patient senses in personnel denial of their terminality he will not attempt to bridge that gap. However, if the patient senses that personnel are willing to deal openly and honestly with him, such as Mrs. Ross sensed from Captain Thomas, the question will be asked.

I shared with staff members the times I became disappointed with certain patients over their apparent reluctance to move towards acceptance of their illness. Only after reflection about our interactions was I able to acknowledge that it was due to my lack of readiness, in most instances, to deal with the subject of death. Each time, the patient would be quick to perceive my reluctance and quickly changed the subject to a neutral topic. Only after I recognized and worked through the reasons for my unreadiness, was I able to again confront the patient and be able to help him.

Sharing these experiences with staff members seemed to strike a response in them as they slowly recalled times when the patient gave them "cues" and they "tuned out." We should not assume that the patient has been told or has not been told about his condition. We need to take our cues from the patient and proceed from there, continually following the patient's pace. What the patient needed to deny yesterday, he may be ready to deal with today.

The remainder of the conference concentrated on identifying Mrs. Ross' needs and how staff members could assist in meeting her needs. One need, manifest to all staff members, was to leave the hospital and stay in Texas with Sandy, her eldest daughter. Staff members felt this could be her "unfinished business" and that Sandy was the daughter she needed to communicate with openly in the short time remaining. Kitty, Mrs. Ross had indicated, would be alright—she had her own internal resources and she did not have to worry about her. How this need might be met posed formidable problems to the staff. Mrs. Ross had been hampered all week by progressive nausea and vomiting. How could she be released to visit her daughter if the nausea and vomiting persisted? Dr. Lyons indicated he planned on inserting a nasogastric tube for draining that afternoon, as well as obtain another GI series to ascertain what might be causing Mrs. Ross' difficulty. They also shared with others certain facts about Mrs. Ross—her need to be as independent as possible. They recognized she would request help if needed, but counted on them to be in the room during the times she would attempt to bathe herself, or get in or out of bed.

The conference ended with staff members determined to meet Mrs. Ross' need to get home to Texas and spend her last few days with her daughter—even if they had to take her to the airport themselves and accompany her to Texas!

During the next few days, Mrs. Ross responded dramatically to tube drainage, resuming all intake with minimal distress. It was during this time that Mrs. Ross showed evidence of increasing discomfort. The area of discomfort was always the same, to the right of the abdominal midline, radiating to spine. She remarked that she no longer was ever free from pain. She did not like to receive pain medication for it seemed to make her "foggy," and she either slept a great deal or, if awake, was unable to think clearly about matters significant to her. Her ability to communicate meaningfully with others, she felt, was markedly reduced at these times and she freely admitted how frightening such experiences were to her.

One day, about a week later, Mrs. Ross remarked to me rather casually, while rubbing her abdomen, "Dr. Lyons seems to think this mass I feel is malignant—Dr. Cairns (another resident) seems to think so too—Dr. Doe is the only one who won't say either way." She looked at me and smiled wanly. Her gaze never left my face. "What do you think the mass is, Mrs. Ross?" "Well, I really think it is malignant—of course I hope Dr. Doe is right when he says it may be from surgical trauma, but I really think it's not." Her hand kept rubbing her abdomen and her face reflected both anguish and pain.

The pain. What could be done about her unrelenting pain. Right now she was sleeping a good deal of the day and most of the night. She remarked that she was unable to do the things she felt she wanted to do because of the drug's "foggy" effect. Yet the current drugs, Demerol and Phenergan, did not relieve the pain. I reviewed her orders and noted she was presently receiving the following medications: Compazine, 10 mg intramuscularly, every 6 hours or as needed for pain; Seconal, 100 mg intramuscularly for sleep, as needed; Tigan suppository, one as needed for nausea; Talwin, one tablet orally every 3 hours or as needed for pain; Demerol, 75 mg intramuscularly, every 4 hours, or as needed for pain; Phenergan, 25 mg intramuscularly, every 4 hours or as needed for pain. I wondered what the chances might be of titrating medications that would relieve her pain, yet keep her mentally alert. I discussed this possibility with Captain Thomas, and described some of the successes we had on other units when the patients became involved in the decision of scheduling their medication. Captain Thomas felt Dr. Doe would be agreeable to such a venture, and planned to talk with him in the morning.

The next day Captain Thomas called and asked me to stop by the unit if I had a moment. When I entered the nursing station, she showed me Mrs. Ross' order sheet signed by Drs. Doe and Lyons. It read: Patient's pain medication is being timed and tested for best results according to her expressed desires. She may receive: Demerol, 25 to 100 mg orally, as needed for pain; Dilaudid, 2 mg orally or intramuscularly, as needed for pain; Percodan tablets, one or two, orally or as needed for pain; Talwin, 50 mg tablets, one or two orally for pain, as needed; Talwin, 30 to 60 mg intramuscularly, as needed for pain; Phenergan, 25 to 50 mg orally or intramuscularly with any of the above medications as needed; Seconal, 100 mg intramuscularly, for sleep, as needed. Drs. Doe and Lyons had stopped by Mrs. Ross' room to briefly explain the new orders. They told her the nurses would fill her in on the details of the new regimen.

Armed with enthusiasm, expectation, and knowledge of the arsenal of medications which could be used to alleviate Mrs. Ross' pain, Captain Thomas and I entered her room to explain her role in this new undertaking.

At first she listened rather passively as we explained the list of medications available to her whenever she expressed her need for them. We captured her undivided attention, however, when we told her we needed her to tell us how effective the drug was that she had requested . . . that we also needed to know any drugs that she had received during this hospitalization that seemed to be more helpful in controlling her pain without making her "foggy."

When we finished, she sat up and slowly repeated all we had said, with special emphasis on: "I can have the medication when I request it?" We reassured her she had understood us correctly. She leaned back in bed and said in a low voice, "It might work, it seems plausible." We suggested she might want to keep a log to record the times she received the medication; the kind she received; if the drug for pain relief was effective, minimally effective, or ineffective; length of time it took to attain pain relief, and how long the drug(s) kept her comfortable. She indicated she would like to keep account of how she felt in a steno notebook. We told her we planned to use her comments in conjunction with the nursing notes to assist in titrating the correct amount of drugs she'd receive. (A comparison of objective observations by nursing staff combined with subjective comments by the patient could be enlightening and useful data now and in the future for this patient as well as others.)

Mrs. Ross asked a few questions about the drugs ordered for her, that is, potency, side effects, and how one drug compared to the other as to dosages ordered. Demerol, she wished to avoid, if at all possible, for this caused her to become "foggy" mentally. Dilaudid, she decided not to use at this time, merely stating, "Let's hold that in abeyance right now." (Although I did not seek validation from her I wondered if use of this powerful narcotic would mean to her that she was much sicker. Right then her need to deny any exaccerbation of illness was paramount, if she was to make it to Texas.)

Mrs. Ross began the new regimen immediately by selecting Percodan. She related that this drug had controlled her pain fairly well in the past and did not have the effect of making her "foggy."

The first day, beginning at 1:40 P.M., Mrs. Ross requested two Percodan tablets, and again at 5 and 9 P.M. She took Seconal, 100 mg at midnight for sleep. Her notes, and those of the nursing staff, revealed that she was fairly comfortable after the second dose of Percodan. She recorded forty minutes as the time required to obtain a fair amount of pain relief. The following day she had the same drug and dosage at 1:45 A.M., 9 A.M., and 3:45 P.M., with notes stating that pain relief was obtained in approximately thirty minutes. Pain was better controlled on the second day, she felt, with only a residual dull pain over her abdomen. Nursing notes revealed that Mrs. Ross appeared more alert and relaxed. She indicated her pleasure and relief at never waiting long for the nurses to bring her medication. It appeared that she was beginning to trust that the nurses would bring her medication without delay. The third day, she requested and received Percodan at 2 A.M, 2 P.M., and 11:30 P.M. The latter dose she decided to combine with 100 mg of Seconal. She awakened the following morning and stated she had no pain! When I visited her several hours later, she looked serene and peaceful. She delighted in sharing the news with all the staff members. For the remainder of her hospital stay, twelve more days, she continued on the above regimen of two tablets of percodan every ten to twelve hours, combining her last dose, before sleeping, with 100 mg of Seconal. She was discharged to visit her relatives in Texas, taking with her the same medications for control of pain. (*Note:* Mrs. Ross lived for fourteen more days, eleven of which were spent with her daughter, Sandy, before requiring further hospitalization. Letters nursing staff received from both daughters after the funeral indicated that Mrs. Ross had indeed been able to complete her "unfinished business.")

• It indeed seems strange that such a system of individualizing patient's pain medication does not occur to us more frequently. There's a strong tendency to become stereotyped in adhering to and perpetuating 3- to 4-hour pain orders when we know that pain differs widely in quality and quantity for each individual. How much more useful to have the patient involved in decision making based on information he gives us to guide us in titrating the degree, duration, and efficacy of medication needed to forestall the onslaught of pain.

A crucial point, I believe, is to stay "on top of the pain," that is, prevent it from ever occurring. This kind of pain control relieves the patient from becoming dependent on clocks and persons administering the drug. It permits him to complete his "unfinished business" without being consumed by pain, or to engage in those pursuits which make his remaining time both satisfying, meaningful, and serene, without the threat of pain.

The control and relief of pain should include the patient. As an active participant–receiver in the titration of pain control, the terminally ill patient knows his request for medication will be acted upon promptly, and that staff members are both interested and involved in the maintenance of pain relief.

He also knows that careful attention and respect will be given to his comments regarding the degree of pain he encounters, and that dosages will be raised or lowered accordingly.

Listening to the patient is often therapeutic in itself—both physical and mental distress can be relieved by being expressed to someone else. One patient summed it up by saying, "In listening, he took part of my pain with him."

A phenomenon noticed while working with terminally ill patients is their frequently voiced need to be "clear and mentally alert." They often elect, if given a choice, to stand moderate and even severe amounts of pain in order to maintain clarity of thought and speech. Pain at that particular time appears to be relegated to a lesser position in the need hierarchy. However, if anti-pain drugs are personalized to relieve the patient's discomfort, yet do not cloud his consciousness, much unnecessary suffering can effectively be avoided. If for some patients this is not possible, nursing personnel, by monitoring the patient's reactions to discomfort, can be respsonive to such variables by rendering anti-pain drugs when the need for alertness and conversation with significant others is less acute.

Although only one experience has been related in personalizing the management of pain for the terminally ill patient, it appears possible to extrapolate the process in personalizing the management of pain for other terminally ill patients.

Personalized care should be the goal for all who are ill, particularly for those in pain. For those who are terminally ill and in pain personalized care must be the norm. Can we be content to settle for less?

Comment

Nurses and physicians obviously used their creative abilities in caring for Mrs. Ross. Although they at first adhered to the usual routine for controlling pain by administering medication every 3 to 4 hours, they eventually moved to another, more innovative and effective way of relieving her pain.

The client was able to participate in her plan of care, was able to make her own decisions, and not only benefitted personally but provided valuable data for personnel who would be able to use this experience to help other clients in similar difficulties. Encouraging independence and providing means by which she could plan her medication regimen to prevent pain made the client more comfortable and was a satisfying experience for personnel who could see the client's physical relief despite the fact that she was being given a reduced amount of medication.

Listening to the client and paying careful attention to her reports on the effects of her medication gave the client a sense of security and firmly reassured her that the personnel involved with her care were interested in her as a person.

This report is a good illustration of the successful way in which health team members can include the client as an active participant in assessing, planning, implementing, and evaluating his care; communication and cooperation are apparent, mutual trust and respect are integral parts of the activity, and the end result is quality care and satisfaction both for the client and for personnel.

• *Situation: Mr. Adam Zappelle in an Intensive Care Unit*

Mr. Zappelle was 65 years old; he really looked younger, despite the ominous appearance of the ventilator at his side, which was making strange noises. The tube that protruded from the newly formed tracheostomy was surely frightening to him, also. The nurse who was just arriving for assignment to the intensive care unit looked briefly at Mr. Zappelle, rapidly assessed those needs that would demand first priority, then went to see what additional information she could obtain about him. She received some data about frequency of medications and the observations to make, but received little data about him as a person. No family members had been seen; no one was available who had personal knowledge about Mr. Zappelle. The record developed by the medical staff suggested he was being treated for an advanced carcinoma of the pharynx, and metastases had been detected in the lymph nodes of the neck. Primary symptoms were pain and an inability to eat because of a poor appetite. The nurse saw an anxious, frightened man with tense, taut muscles. In addition to the up-and-down motion and the sound of the ventilator bellows, sounds of the cardiac monitor added to the usual bustle of activity in such a unit. To provide further discomfort for Mr. Zappelle, a Foley catheter was in place, an intravenous infusion was running, and his arm was stabilized to an armboard to prevent him from moving it. These areas of assessment were apparent; no one could miss these in any review of client needs. The astute nurse had just arrived to care for the acutely ill persons on this unit and saw beyond Mr. Zappelle's obvious problems. As she spoke to him and introduced herself, he looked at her with eyes that seemed to reveal many messages. The nurse could not read all of the unvoiced messages, but she inferred he needed some comfort, some respect for himself as a person, some relief from many physical restrictions, some ease in breathing, and some understanding of what he was enduring.

The nurse decided that one of his major needs, at this point, was to communicate; his vital signs were stabilized sufficiently, the ventilator was helping his breathing problem, but his fear was still very obvious. Perhaps if he could communicate with someone and share his fears, the nurse and others on the medical and nursing teams could plan to cope with his problems. The nurse decided to suggest to him that he use a pencil and paper to tell her what he wanted and the things he wanted to say, because he could not express himself verbally. He was informed that the nurse would spend 10 to 15 minutes out of every 2 hours just talking with him, discussing the equipment around him, explaining its purposes and helping him to understand the medical therapy being planned for him.

Surely it was not the nurse's imagination, but Mr. Zappelle seemed to relax a bit after being told the nurse would visit him regularly. The visits with the nurse were profitable and revealing. She confirmed her suspicions that Mr. Zappelle was accustomed to being very independent. Obviously, being confined to bed in an intensive care unit was not conducive to independence. The next challenge to the nurse was to determine the activities in which he could become involved to assume some of his own care. Gradually he learned to care for the Foley catheter, learned to suction the mucus from his mouth, and became more able to turn himself at regular intervals as the intravenous infusions were reduced and finally eliminated. En-

> couraged by his increasing ability to care for himself his appetite for food returned; he began to eat better, selected foods he liked and preferred, and generally took on the glow of successful recovery. Although his progress to complete recovery would be prolonged, it was in a positive direction, promising to all but especially to Mr. Zappelle.

Comment

Assessment of obvious problems as well as subtle or covert needs is important in all care. Many of both types of problems were present in this situation and an astute nurse observed some discrete behaviors. The challenge of communicating with one who cannot speak was solved by planning new and different approaches to communication, and by implementing them. The client's obvious progression to a unit that was not an acute care area undoubtedly suggests that the approaches used by those caring for Mr. Zappelle were successful. The fact that he progressed to a point where he could assume increased responsibility for his own care also illustrates the effectiveness of these approaches.

The nurse was sensitive to the fact that Mr. Zappelle had lost his ability to communicate verbally; coping with such a handicap, whether it is temporary or permanent, necessitates a totally new body image construct. By carefully assessing the client's condition, the nurse can determine action that can be supportive to him.

• *Situation: Sally Sillick in an Adolescent Unit of a General Hospital*

The adolescent years can be a serious time of life for a 15-year-old; it can be quite complicated when this growing-up phase includes coping with possible rheumatic fever.

> When Sally Sillick was admitted to the adolescent unit of a general hospital, she complained of a very red, swollen, hot-to-touch, and painful left knee. Extensive examinations and tests established the diagnosis; careful observation for possible symptoms of carditis was done conscientiously. Immediate therapy included strict bed rest and a course of salicylates. Within 24 hours, the tenderness and swelling in her knee had subsided, but all other evidence confirmed the diagnosis of rheumatic fever. Treatment was to be prolonged and trying

for this young girl, and her reaction to the diagnosis and proposed treatment was to withdraw.

Sally's mother was very attentive; she came to the hospital each day and spent many hours talking with Sally, reading to her, and exerting every effort to find something to stimulate her interest. Although her mother chatted with other young girls in the four-bed room, Sally showed no interest in joining any of the conversations. In fact, when the others tried to get her to socialize, she crawled deeper under the covers, making it clear to her peers and to her mother that she would not socialize with them. Watching television was her only interest; she would not read fiction, let alone any of her school texts. Soon, there was evidence that she was not eating, although she did agree to take medications brought to her, and permitted nursing personnel to check her vital signs and involve her in the necessary activities of personal hygiene. The nurse who was responsible for Sally's care was quite concerned, however, and she could not think of any approach different from that which she had already used to try to get through to Sally and overcome her obvious withdrawal behavior.

To try to find a different approach to Sally, the nurse assigned to her care asked that the next conference be devoted to Sally's problems as well as those confronting the nurse who was trying to provide her care. A discussion of Sally's behavior led to the suggestion that she may be experiencing some deeper anxiety that she had not yet expressed verbally. The diagnoses of withdrawal, refusal to eat, unwillingness to socialize, and lack of motivation were not difficult to define, but it was difficult to assess the underlying cause of these diagnoses. The group members suggested that the nurse who cared for Sally should pursue different topics of conversation than she had used in the past to find one that would evoke some reaction from Sally.

Armed with some new ideas from her group conference, the nurse mentally preplanned various topics she would introduce to Sally, and several of the subjects had to do with girls' hobbies. A slight spark of interest was kindled when the nurse mentioned knitting. She pursued this topic cautiously, trying, in a judicious manner, to restrain her joy, hoping that the slight interest she had evoked might be broadened into a healthy one.

Returning to the conference room that afternoon, the nurse assigned to Sally's care gave a hopeful report, and the group, now acting as consultants to the nurse, provided her with another idea to suggest to Sally. One of the children in the pediatric unit on the next floor was anxious to have one of the new knitted sweaters that so many of the children were wearing, but the child's mother could not afford to buy her one. Would it be possible to ask the child's mother to buy some yarn and, at the strategic time, ask Sally to knit a sweater for the little child? When the nurse followed through with this suggestion, Sally brightened and showed obvious enthusiasm for the first time since she was hospitalized. The nurses were pleased, and Sally's mother was happy and grateful for the apparent progress in Sally's attitude toward her illness and her required restrictions.

Unfortunately, Sally's enthusiasm for knitting was short-lived. Just about a week after plans had been made for her to knit the sweater, the nurse came into the room after the physicians had been in to visit and found Sally lying very quietly in bed, staring out the window. A cheerful greeting from the nurse brought no response, and it was apparent that she had lapsed into the same type of withdrawal she had experienced previously. The nurse attempted to talk about knitting the sweater, but Sally did not respond. Abruptly, the nurse said, "Sally, are you afraid?" Sally burst into tears, and in the next hour, amid tears and sobs, she told the nurse how frightened she was of the "heart condition" she had, and how she knew she would never be able to do what other girls her age could do. The nurse was surprised to learn that this was Sally's perception of her illness, when in fact, her prognosis for complete recovery, with no residual, was very good.

As soon as the nurse was able to do so, she called the attending physician and discussed the events of the day with him. He promptly called Sally's mother to discuss the incident with her and to correct any misinformation she had about the illness. When the physician came to see Sally and talked with her about what she could expect and how hopeful she could be, Sally became an entirely different person. She became more cheerful, had a healthier appetite, and became more interested in her environment and in those around her.

Comment

It can be assumed that Sally experienced an uneventful recovery after it was discovered she had been misinformed about her illness and the misinformation was corrected. The astute observations of the nurse in assessing withdrawal symptoms and her willingness to discuss and consult with her peers to get ideas and suggestions are all positive aspects of the nursing process. The nurse continued to evaluate each of the approaches she used to find a better or different way to provide for Sally's needs; she was keenly aware of

Sally's varying moods and her reactions to the techniques used to provide the necessary care. Collaboration with the attending physician reinforced the nurse's role in sharing information with related health care workers; the physician's prompt response suggests he appreciated the nurse's alertness to the propitious moment to ask pertinent questions abruptly. Different phases of the nursing process and the different roles assumed by health care personnel on the health team can be identified in this situation.

• *Situation: Mr. Seehew in an Intensive Care Unit*

Mr. I. Seehew was 52 years old when he underwent surgery for the repair of a dissecting aneurysm. He was admitted to the intensive care unit as a critically ill person whose life-sustaining equipment included a respirator, an endotracheal tube, chest tubes, urinary bladder catheter, and intravenous equipment. He had experienced gastric bleeding and convulsions, and by the second week, postoperatively, he had not yet regained consciousness. Even though the life-sustaining equipment was removed, his vital signs remained stable.

Because he was in the unit for an extended period of time, the nursing staff was becoming "insensitive" to Mr. Seehew's needs and the nurses' reaction to him was becoming negative. His prognosis was apparently negative and the nurses who were tuned to caring for more acutely ill persons were rebelling at the idea of caring for this person who was stabilized although still acutely ill, and who did not require the kind of care nurses were accustomed to give in the "intensive, insensitive, expensive" unit. That the nurses rejected the client was apparent. Mrs. Seehew was his only relative and she became aware of the staff's feelings toward her husband. The nursing supervisor was informed about the situation by concerned nursing and medical staff members, and a meeting of the nurses was called to discuss the situation.

Through discussion, skillfully guided by the supervisor, the nurses' feelings about the client were revealed and explored. The revelation was not too surprising, and the nursing staff members should have been sensitive to what was going on before the meeting was called. However, it is sometimes necessary for a chain of events to occur before anyone becomes fully aware of what is happening in such a situation. The usual goal in the intensive care unit is to care for the client's immediate physiologic needs; nurses in the unit are especially skilled in the technical care of the critically ill. Because Mr. Seehew had remained in the unit for a longer period of time than is usual for most patients, most of the care for his physiologic needs was fairly well routinized. Having met these needs, the nurses should have proceeded to fulfill his other needs, but failed to recognize them. They were not consciously aware that their own behavior was contributing to Mr. Seehew's inadequate care. Also, the nurses had overlooked the needs of the client's wife, who was going through a period of stress and crisis. Caring for and being aware of her psychologic needs were just as important as meeting Mr. Seehew's needs.

At the end of the group discussion, a number of questions were raised and the nurses tried to answer their own inquiries. As a result of their self-examination, the following set of objectives was defined:

1. Discuss Mr. Seehew's plan of care with the medical staff to get information about the medical plan and to share the goals of the nursing plan.
2. Identify his level of physiologic needs and establish other needs the nurses can help to meet.
3. Establish a plan of caring for the client's wife and help her to meet her needs in a way similar to the plan being established for Mr. Seehew.

The nurses set these as the immediate, short-range goals; they knew that other, long-range goals would soon be necessary, but immediate goals were the most important now, for the benefit of the client and to motivate and stimulate the interest of the staff nurses.

Each nurse on the staff of the unit felt deeply committed to accomplish the goals that had been established by the nursing group for the benefit of Mr. Seehew. Each nurse supported the other in her efforts to achieve the established goals. Communication between the medical staff and the nursing staff improved; each seemed to compete with the other to achieve the best performance in taking care of Mr. Seehew. His wife responded positively to the increased concern demonstrated by the nurses; the staff's pleasure grew as they saw the success of their efforts.

Within seven days from the time of the conference, Mr. Seehew was transferred to another unit in the hospital; a complete report of all his needs and the nursing care plan that was so successful while he was in the intensive care unit was shared with nurses who would now be caring for him. One month after he was transferred from the intensive care unit, Mr. Seehew regained consciousness. Sometime later, he was able to walk in his room and to function independently. His recovery was attributed to the success of the staff in assessing his and their needs, to their cooperative planning, to implementing a plan that was shared cooperatively between medicine and nursing and later with other disciplines on the health team, as well as to the constant reassessment of established goals.

Comment

The success of the endeavor illustrated above depends largely on the honesty of the nursing staff with each other and the degree to which they have established mutual trust and respect. Willingness to reveal their true feelings about caring for a client is usually not spontaneous. When one has become caught in a routine that is obviously depersonalizing, conscious awareness of this error is not attractive to those involved. Nurses are to be commended when they use appropriate avenues to discuss what has happened to the process of client care when they realize it has or is threatening to deteriorate. Including the soul-searching self-assessment, as did these nurses in this situation, is commendable.

• *Situation: Miss Lott in a General Hospital*

To carry out the nursing process with a client whose culture is different from that of the nurse presents quite a challenge. To better understand the behaviors of the client, Mona Lott, the nurse had to learn as much as possible about a different culture, to communicate in as many ways as possible with the client and her family, and to use all of her ingenuity and available resources to influence members of the nursing and hospital staff to go along with the suggested plan. The results were gratifying to the nurse and were appreciated by the recipients—the client and her family.

Some of the nurse's observations on Mona were direct; others were indirect. But, all observations contributed to increasing her knowledge about what illness means to the Navajo. Essentially, illness means that something is out of harmony—out of tune with nature. The Navajo believes that only the medicine man can cure illness; the white man's doctor can treat only symptoms. The medicine man tries to remove the evil that has caused the illness; the white man cannot do this. Mona was convinced that as soon as some of her symptoms were treated at the hospital, she would be allowed to return to her home where a ritual could be performed to make her well.

An assessment of her status convinced the nurse that Mona was losing her hope of getting well; she was beginning to despair of experiencing the ritual that would make her well.

Goals were directed to encourage hope; to accomplish this,

another objective was necessary: some arrangements had to be made for the ritual. A major hurdle was to convince the hospital administrators that this ritual was necessary for the welfare and eventual recovery of the client. The hurdles proved to be surmountable, and arrangements were made to have the ritual performed in the hospital room.

To all who observed the abbreviated form of the ritual it was a tremendous experience. The actual rite was shorter than usual because it was performed in the hospital. Essentials of the rite were included, however, and we could see that efforts to arrange for the ritual were successful. It was not long before Mona began to respond to the treatment of the white man's doctor. Because she believed the evil that had caused her illness was removed by the medicine man's ritual, she now had a more positive outlook toward recovery. With renewed hope, Mona responded to medications so promptly that her recovery was phenomenal. The nurses had assessed the primary problem Mona was experiencing and were able to plan and implement methods to cope successfully with the diagnosed problem. From the data gathered by means of observation, it was concluded that the efforts were sucessful. Knowledge, decisions, judgment, and collaboration with members of the health team and the client's family were all directed toward the desirable outcome for the client.

Comment

This example shows the importance of coping with that problem most important to the client. All of the treatment and medications the client had received were of no benefit as long as she believed the source of her illness, or evil, was still present in her body. By providing the only person she believed could remove the evil, the health team was able to provide treatment that helped her to recover; the client's psychologic and physical states were responsive because she was receptive. This report also illustrates the major role culture plays in working with and caring for people. Each person responds as a total unit to others in his environment; the physical, psychosocial, and cultural components of an individual blend harmoniously into one.

• *Situation: Mrs. Russe in a General Hospital*

Mrs. Vi Russe was hospitalized for several weeks. Her problem was chronic herpes zoster, and medication was not controlling the pain. Mrs. Russe was taught to administer her own medication; her husband was involved in the instruction sessions, and both seemed anxious to have Vi at home again. Despite the apparent success of all treatments, Vi's condition did not progress as it should have or as it was expected to.

To determine the reason for stabilization in less than a positive state, records were scoured for clues; conferences were held with various health team members; and discussions were conducted with Mrs. Russe and her husband. Finally, when all data were assembled and analyzed, it was found that Mrs. Russe had regressed from a relative independent state to one of dependence; however, no real cause for the regression could be determined.

Conferences were held by the nursing staff members; the goal was to try to ascertain why the client's need for help in providing for her daily needs had increased and why her ambulation and socialization had decreased. To obtain some answers to these questions, the same nurse was assigned to her care as frequently as possible. The plan included frequent visits, a positive, friendly manner, and communication by word and action that people were interested in her; nurses were to be alert for any clues that might present themselves, and they were to encourage independence. Despite deliberate planning to meet these goals, only minimal results were achieved.

Evaluation and replanning led to a new approach. Less emphasis would be placed on independence; her state of dependence would be accepted; discussion of matters such as the dangers of prolonged bedrest would be limited; all these would be pursued while trying to anticipate and provide for as many of Mrs. Russe's needs as could be determined. After several days in which this latter approach was used, an evaluation conference revealed that Mrs. Russe was responding well to this indirect approach. She appeared to be taking more interest in her own care and expressed some desire to get out of bed more often. On several occasions she responded to conversation initiated by the other client in the room; this was something she had not done before. Gradually, she responded to treatment sufficiently to be discharged. She was still dependent on others for some assistance, but there was some movement toward increasing independence. The medical and nursing staff members concluded that Mrs. Russe was now sufficiently motivated to continue her positive progress. Follow-up visits at her home are needed to confirm this conclusion.

Comment

Although not presented in complete detail in terms of medications, treatment, or all of the problems with which Mrs. Russe had to cope, this report suggests that the approach to planning and implementing any plan of care should be thoroughly individualized. The approach that was used for one client may not be effective for another. Some clients resent, whereas others respond well to, a direct approach. It is important for the nurse to read clues as well as she can and to make decisions and judgments based on her knowledge of human behavior to determine the approach she should use in any one situation.

• *Situation: Mr. Zdroak in a General Hospital*

Mr. Zdroak had a cerebral vascular accident on Thursday. By Saturday morning his semicomatose state cleared. When the nurse entered his room he was sobbing; his left arm and leg were limp and motionless at his side.

The nursing process was triggered by the nurse's perception of the client's behavior; she assessed the client's state as discomfort and depression. She inferred that he was frustrated, frightened, and helpless to cope with his situation. The nurse's goal was to share with him her perception of his state, determine whether her perceptions were correct, and explore what this experience means to him. To initiate the conversation, the nurse said, "I know you are concerned about being unable to move your arm and your leg." The client replied, "Yes, I am very upset about it. My brother had the same thing happen to him some 5 years ago and he was helpless for 2 years before he died. I thought it just could not happen to me, but it has happened. I just don't want to become as helpless as my brother."

This response from Mr. Zdroak validated the nurse's perception, but she also found the reason for his concern—he had seen his brother in a similar state. The nurse, by her presence, by her well-phrased questions, by permitting appropriate pauses and silences during the conversation, communicated to Mr. Zdroak that she was interested in him as a person, was concerned about his fears, and was willing and available to help him during the recovery process. Although some of the communication was nonverbal, the client responded positively to the nurse's approach. She was formulating judgments and making decisions while she was communicating with him and identifying his most immediate need—help in coping with his frustration and despair—so that a rehabilitation program could be implemented. Gradually, the client began to accept the nurse, saw that she was willing to help him, and a beginning trust was established, which would grow and develop over a period of time.

The short-range goal was to begin a program of therapy for the client's paralyzed arm and leg. The nurse shared with him the plan of exercise and activity advised for him. He reacted by comparing the exercise program with one he had used on his farm: "We only exercise the animals' legs after they are injured, if we think they will be able to use them again." No doubt Mr. Zdroak thought, "Maybe I'll be able to walk again." After thinking for awhile about the idea of exercise, the client stroked his left hand and arm and said, "There is no feeling, but they are warm; they are alive; maybe those exercises will help. I'll move my good arm and leg, and if you will help me move the other arm and leg, maybe I can do something besides stay in this bed, lying flat on my back." The communication from Mr. Zdroak told the nurse that he was receptive to exercise; he even suggested a way to implement the exercise plan.

The nurse eagerly picked up the cue the client provided, and gave him necessary instructions about how to exercise and how long to continue his effort so that he would not overtire himself.

Throughout the entire effort, the nurse encouraged the client to perform the exercise program and she continually evaluated his response to the activity. She continued to listen to him to pick up any cues that would suggest further acceptance of his true state, or to indicate any regression in attitude or physical state.

Mr. Zdroak's behavior throughout the exercise program validated the nurse's assumption that he associated exercise with recovery. His behavior told the staff members that he was no longer preoccupied with fear and pessimism but saw himself as increasingly capable of handling the demands of his situation, because he had been given the necessary help when he was physically unable to help himself.

Comment

The importance of accurate assessment cannot be overemphasized. Careful and astute observation of crucial parameters is essential. It is also important for the nurse to validate her observations with the client. Does the nurse view symptoms and behavior only from her own perspective, or does she seek ways to communicate with the client to confirm the accuracy of her assessment? Having established the problem areas that are of major concern to the client, the nurse uses the cues he provides to develop a plan of care that will help him to cope with the problems identified. Because the goals of care were established by the mutual efforts of nurse and client, the evaluation phase of the process can proceed in an orderly, systematic manner.

• *Situation: Mr. Elder in a Nursing Home*

Mr. Elder was about 90 years old; he had muscle contractures of the knees, hips, elbows, shoulders, as well as extensive decubiti of the sacrum and lateral thigh. He had difficulty swallowing food, and was becoming malnourished because no one spent enough time to feed him. They did not have the time to wait until he coped with dysphagia sufficiently to get some food into his stomach. When a new nurse was transferred to the area where Mr. Elder was located, he was one of the first clients for whom a conference was scheduled. His multiple problems made it obvious that Mr. Elder needed some very special care. The nurses discussed the probable cause of the decubiti and concluded that he was turned from side-to-side infrequently; hence prolonged periods of lying in one position could easily cause decubiti to develop. A malnourished state fostered skin ulcerations and abrasions in multiple areas of his body. Problems experienced by Mr. Elder were identified as:

1. Decubiti needed immediate attention and care.
2. Dietary intake was poor in quantity and quality.
3. Mr. Elder was hard of hearing.
4. There was no apparent means of sensory stimulation.
5. Attitude of staff nurses was "why worry about bedsores when he is so sick he probably cannot live too long anyhow."
6. Because of the multiple care needs, more than one person should be assigned to care for him.

After these were identified as major problem areas, another session was held to determine the best way to cope with them.

Planning was done chiefly by the professional nurse at first, but her secondary aim was to motivate other nursing personnel to see Mr. Elder in a more positive way, to see his potential for relative recovery, and to implement measures of care, using their own initiative.

A 20-minute turning schedule was set, with two team members assigned to turn Mr. Elder at scheduled times. His right and left sides and abdomen were used in turning him, and he was never placed on his back because the decubiti on the sacrum were severe. Each time he was turned, the decubiti were washed, dried, and ointment was applied. A heat lamp was used regularly to promote drying and the tissue was treated very cautiously. These measures gradually were successful. Feeding was planned at short intervals, using small amounts of food with a high protein content, such as custards, soft cooked eggs, eggnog, and a special protein feeding.

A discussion of nurses' attitudes about caring for older people and the importance of taking care of the "living" rather than the "dying" person eventually made an impact on personnel. After a deliberate and continued instruction session with nursing aides, they began to spend more time with Mr. Elder, took the necessary time to feed him, turn him, and, eventually, to be patient enough to speak slowly and distinctly so that shouting at the hard-of-hearing Mr. Elder was no longer necessary. Communication was finally effective. After seven days of discussion and prodding by the head nurse, the decubiti were dry and granulation tissue had begun to appear around the edges of the ulcerated area. Mr. Elder began to respond by speaking to those around him more often. His increased dietary intake was beginning to show effects: he had more energy, became more alert, and was making more demands for attention. These evidences of progress stimulated the staff; they could see the results of their efforts and began to work harder to try to accomplish more. It was now a challenge to them to see who could do the most for Mr. Elder. There was still a long way to go to full recovery, but the first steps had been taken.

Comment

Introducing a new face and some fresh ideas into a fairly stabilized situation can be a threat to personnel or it can produce qualitative results.

The newly assigned nurse described in this situation was a person-oriented practitioner who recognized the dignity of Mr. Elder and who visualized the constructive efforts that could be made on his behalf. Having the courage to lead personnel who had fallen into a routine of care in a different direction is not easy. It is essential and important, however, when the client's welfare is the ultimate goal. Using instrumental as well as expressive roles, this nurse effectively directed the staff toward assessing Mr. Elder's problems carefully, and to use initiative and originality in planning and implementing the care he required. Evaluation in terms of improved physical status is quite apparent; more subtle areas of providing sensory stimulation, for example, require more discreet measures.

• *Situation: Mrs. Fida in the Hospital and at Home*

Mrs. B.I. Fida is a 28-year-old multipara. She had come to the hospital entrance, obviously in active labor, although her expected date of delivery was 4 weeks away. Diagnostic examinations had previously confirmed twins. Despite premature labor, she progressed normally through the different stages, and 8 hours after she was admitted to the labor room, she delivered twin boys. One boy, Twin A., weighed just less than 4 pounds and was normal in appearance. The other boy, Twin B., weighed just over 4 pounds and appeared to have possible mild hydrocephalus.

A spontaneous cry from each boy at birth brought the usual smile of joy to personnel in the delivery room. As could be expected, it was not very long before the mother asked anxiously, "Are they all right?" A very brief delay was evident before Mrs. Fida's question was answered. The doctor moved to her side after he completed a cursory examination of the infants, and with deep and sincere compassion, couched his words into the type of phrases that would tell the mother she had borne twin boys; one appeared quite normal, but the other appeared to have mild hydrocephalus. Mrs. Fida had a great deal of confidence in her physician, and her trust in his truthfulness was apparent; she cried and was obviously distressed at the information she had received, but she seemed to cling to the careful use of the word "mild" hydrocephalus. The doctor promised Mrs. Fida he would see her in a few hours, after she had time to recover from the effects of some of the medications. He promised to spend as much time as she wished, talking about the children. Though the mother's disappointment was still very obvious, she appeared satisfied with the doctor's explanation and his promise to come back to discuss the babies' welfare very soon.

When the doctor left the delivery room, Mrs. Fida asked the nurse if she could see the babies. The incubators were moved close enough for her to see the infants, and the nurse raised Mrs. Fida's shoulders and head so she could look at the newborn boys. When she was no longer able to keep her shoulders and head raised from the table, Mrs. Fida laid her head back on the arms of the nurse and sobbed gently; the nurse stood silently, then gradually lowered Mrs. Fida's head as her sobs began to subside. Words were not important now, nor were they necessary at this stage. The mere presence of the nurse, holding Mrs. Fida's hand, and communicating by her facial expression and touch that she understood and sympathized, was all that was necessary at the moment.

The doctor stood at the delivery room door with Mr. Fida, and together the doctor and nurse told him the news and showed him the babies, as they had the mother. Mr. Fida, too, was tearful and disappointed. The doctor and nurse left the room at that time so that mother and father could be alone to share the grief and disappointment that always accompanies the birth of a less than normal child.

While the parents were grappling with their reactions to this event and trying to cope with their feelings, the nurse was having a similar problem. She felt it was necessary for her to acknowledge her own reactions to the birth of such a child, and to be aware of her feelings of disappointment, certainly different in caliber than those of the parents but, nevertheless, very real. Her immediate impulse was to retreat, to remove herself from the area, but this was a fleeting thought. Actually, she knew she would care for the mother, and deliberately began to plan the way to approach that care. She decided she would show interest in both children, she would provide every possible opportunity for mother and father to discuss their feelings about the twins with her, especially Twin B., who had hydrocephalus. Also, the nurse obtained as much information as she could that would be useful to the Fida family, and planned to make opportunities available for them to see other parents who had successfully coped with children who were born with similar handicaps. Above all, the nurse and the doctor were convinced of the importance of being honest with the parents, and the parents knew they could depend on the forthrightness of these two persons. Having established their trust and confidence in the physician and the nurse, Mr. and Mrs. Fida had taken the first major step in the long road to adjusting to their new role, that of being the parents of a handicapped child.

As the normal twin progressed in his feedings, and his weight increased, Mrs. Fida became more encouraged; gradually the nurse involved Mrs. Fida in the feeding activity, and this was especially helpful in raising her morale. Initially, the infant feeding was somewhat difficult for the mother; apparently she would think more vividly, at each feeding, about the other twin who was not on the same feeding schedule. Before long, the nurse included the mother in Twin B.'s feeding schedule too, bringing her in to observe the infant feeding. As the mother became more assured of the baby's ability to take the feedings, she was more confident of her own abilities, and assisted with feeding both babies in a short time.

Both babies reached a fairly stable state, and Mrs. Fida had sufficiently recovered so that she was ready to be discharged from the hospital. Two children at home, one in the fourth grade at school and one in the first grade, concerned the parents; how would they react to the new baby who was "different?" The parents were encouraged to discuss with the children the fact that the new babies would be coming home later, and that one of the babies was different from most. The children were encouraged by the parents that they would be able to work together as a family to help the new babies, especially Twin B. The approach to these discussions was a positive one, stressing the valuable opportunity available to the family to care for such a special child.

Having coped with discussing the new babies with the children at home, the parents were faced with another challenge—the reactions of relatives and friends. When the parents verbally expressed their concerns about these reactions, the nurse encouraged them to continue their positive approach to the twins, and operate on the premise that their positive and matter-of-fact attitude and manner would become a role model for observant relatives and friends. Instructions to the parents were realistic; they were told that the course of events would not be totally smooth; there would be times the parents would be discouraged, and there would be occasions when it would be most difficult to put up a positive front. To cope with such occasions, the nurse and doctor provided the parents with names, addresses, and phone numbers of some professional persons who would be available to them when they found it difficult to cope with the problem. They were also given the name of a parents' organization where they could meet others caring for exceptional children.

The Fida children were eagerly waiting for their mother to return home from the hospital; to the parents' relief, they did not seem worried that one of their brothers would be "different." (Such is the innocence of youth.) Between the day Mrs. Fida returned from the hospital and the day the twins were brought home, many hours were spent in talking with the children about their responsibilities when the new babies came home. The youngsters were equal to the task before them, and Mr. and Mrs. Fida began to settle slowly into a more comfortable role than they thought would be possible.

The first encounter with close relatives was not nearly so traumatic as the parents feared it would be—perhaps because they had succeeded so well in developing their own abilities to cope with the situation and in preparing the children for the new babies' arrival. Not all days were smooth, and suggested resources were used on numerous occasions. However, all were coping with the situation and were making constructive efforts to support Mr. and Mrs. Fida in every possible way.

Comment

The emotionally laden event of the birth of a handicapped child poses major challenges to personnel who care for the child and/or the parents involved. This situation illustrates how important it is for the nurse to be aware of her own feelings and reactions, essentially assessing her own needs and problem areas before she will be able to help the clients for whom she is responsible. Conscious, deliberate assessment and determination of ways to cope with acknowledged assets and limitations are essential steps in the process of planning for the care of the client who needs some professional assistance.

The care process illustrated in this situation initially takes place in the hospital, but the nurse moved beyond the immediate situation to plan ways in which the client could cope with anticipated problems in the home setting. Forecasting and predicting are not essentials of nursing, but assuming and hypothesizing are innate qualities that contribute to the level of performance of the nurse. Astute listening to the client's fears and concerns as she prepares to go home from the hospital will provide the nurse with cues that can help her to plan with the client for anticipated eventualities. Follow-up visits by the nurse to the home, or return visits of the client to the hospital or clinic make data available from which the effectiveness of the planning in preparation for the return to the home can be determined.

• *Situation: Mrs. R. N. Lombardo in a General Hospital*

Mrs. R.N. Lombardo is a nurse who has home, family, and professional responsibilities. She is a forty-year-old widow with two teen-aged children, a boy and a girl, both of whom are in high school. Since her husband's death five years ago, she has been employed in a large, active, outpatient department of the city hospital and last year she assumed the head nurse position. A gregarious person by nature, she enjoys having people and activity in her environment most of the time.

While pursuing her household chores last week, Mrs. Lombardo experienced an acute episode of low back pain. After being examined by her personal physician, she was admitted to a medical and surgical unit of the hospital where she is employed. X-rays revealed a degenerative disc. Conservative measures were initiated, but the pain has not been alleviated to any appreciable degree.

The nursing staff are very fond of Mrs. Lombardo and they have exerted a great deal of effort to help her obtain relief from the pain. Her anxiety has become more marked as it becomes apparent that her pain is not responding to the conservative treatment. Mrs. Lombardo is resisting the idea of surgery; she feels it will take her away from her responsibilities for too long a time. Despite the availability of some accumulated sick leave and the willingness of her sister to stay with her daughter and son while Mrs. Lombardo is hospitalized, she feels an obligation to resume her own roles as soon as possible.

The knowledge of the disc pathology along with the extensive discussions with her physician have not impressed her with the need for surgery as the preferred treatment. Each day Mrs. Lombardo's appetite decreases; she rejects the usual diet that she previously enjoyed, and even the frequent telephone conversations with her children and her sister are not as pleasant and positive in tone as they were at the beginning of the week.

Sensing some urgency in arriving at a definitive plan for Mrs. Lombardo, the clinical specialist on the unit arranged for a nursing conference about Mrs. Lombardo. They concluded that her primary problems were actual pain, fear of increasing and continued pain, and anxiety about fulfilling her responsibilities. Realizing that one week is a relatively short period of time to determine the effectiveness of the conservative therapy, it was decided that the goals of the nursing staff would be:

1. Continue the conservative therapy for one more week.
2. Have the clinical specialist spend some time each morning and afternoon with Mrs. Lombardo discussing the expected outcomes of the conservative therapy and compare these to the expected outcomes of the surgery. By doing this, the clinical specialist reinforces the discussions and explanation provided for Mrs. Lombardo by her physician and by the nursing staff.
3. Discuss with the physician the possibility of Mrs. Lombardo returning to her home and continuing on the conservative therapy program at home. In the home setting she could resume some parts of her role as head of the family, and as a mother. Evidence suggests the son and daughter would be supportive of their mother at home.
4. Involve Mrs. Lombardo in the decision making about the setting where the therapy would be most effective—at home, or in the hospital; assist her in setting time limits for the conservative treatment so that an extensive time period will not be devoted to meaningless therapy. Assist Mrs. Lombardo to conclude that at the end of the agreed upon time period for conservative treatment, if improvement is not apparent, then the surgery can be considered for correction of the disc problem.

The nursing plans for Mrs. Lombardo will proceed according to the defined goals. At the end of each day, the clinical specialist and the nursing staff will review each goal and will, in collaboration with Mrs. Lombardo, determine whether any progress has been made. If some changes have occurred, the goals will be redefined as necessary, and care will continue as it has been done during the past week, or indicated changes will be made.

Comment

The nurses who were responsible for Mrs. Lombardo's care were able to define three major needs, namely, freedom from pain, from fear, and from anxiety. Obviously, Mrs. Lombardo had other problems, such as anorexia, and other needs, such as mobility, elimination, electrolyte balance, socialization, etc. Establishing the need priority is the legitimate means of defining care goals. Once the more crucial needs are coped with, other needs become primary and are defined and focused on as the care plan is periodically revised.

One factor that underlies the care of Mrs. Lombardo is the fact that she is a nurse who has occupied a leadership position in nursing. The expectations that the nursing staff hold about her should be explored to ascertain whether the feelings of the staff are affecting the care of Mrs. Lombardo. The clinical specialist may need to seek psychologic consultation to determine to what extent the nurses have feelings toward and about Mrs. Lombardo. Some nurses experience very positive feelings about an ill coworker, whereas others are threatened by or feel insecure in caring for such a person in a patient role. Other nurses may hold unreasonable expectations of Mrs. Lombardo; that is, because she is a nurse, she should have certain knowledge and behavior, and these should be different from other clients' knowledge and behavior. The clinical specialist can assume the role of coordinator of Mrs. Lombardo's care and assist the staff in the continual assessment of themselves as well as periodically and regularly reviewing the status of Mrs. Lombardo's needs.

• *Situation: Mr. Paul Z. Mhuto at Home*

Let me introduce myself: My name is Paul, and I have lived in this youth and health-oriented society for 53 years as a victim of athetoid type cerebral palsy. It is speculated that an impatient obstetrician delivered me by forceps, despite the fact I was born two months prematurely and my mother had delivered a nine-pound baby two years previously with no difficulty. At six months of age I contracted a "polio-like" childhood illness that was never clearly diagnosed, but there was no question about the aftermath of the illness: my right leg was never to develop fully and my hearing was totally lost.

Life was not unkind to me because my parents, siblings, relatives, and friends were kind; they recognized my handicaps but permitted me to utilize my available strengths to the maximum. Schools for the deaf prepared me for reading and writing and, despite the palsy, for carpentry, which I have followed successfully. The stares of strangers have been tolerated these 53 years with varying degrees of patience.

Two years ago, a routine physical examination revealed hypertension, which is being successfully controlled with Dyazide. Six months ago I developed numbness and tingling in my fingers and toes. Within two months from the onset of this sensory alteration, I began to have difficulty in walking. Within three and a half months, I was using a cane; in four months, the walker was necessary for ambulation. At the end of five months, I found I was able to move about only with the aid of a wheelchair and the fine movements of my fingers were diminished. I was now unable to accomplish the activities of daily living that I had been able to accomplish independently during these past five decades—I now needed someone to assist me. Despite numerous diagnostic tests, no medical diagnosis was established.

Let me introduce myself: I am Nurse Em Dobra who has known Paul for a number of years; I have assumed the challenge of assisting Paul's family to help them and him to cope with Paul's needs.

The primary need for *food and fluids* is provided by Paul's brother's family, with whom he lives. Prior to six months ago, Paul prepared his own breakfast and lunch in his own living quarters, then joined the family in their home for dinner. Now, Paul is dependent on his relatives to bring breakfast and lunch to him; he is then wheeled in the wheelchair to his brother's home for dinner. Between meal fluids are available in his own kitchen; the refrigerator is placed so that he can wheel to the door and obtain cool drinks as needed.

Comment

This provides for the essential intake of food and fluids. Apparently the nutrition status is being maintained adequately. What psychological effect does this altered living pattern have on Paul? How does he perceive himself now, having to be dependent on others for food when he was relatively independent for many years? Does he enjoy the attention? Does he resent his inability to be independent? Is he motivated to try to walk again? Is there a change in th socialization patterns at meal-times? What effect would or could such changes have on Paul? on his family? Does the family resent taking meals to him at breakfast and at lunch?

Elimination

With the assistance of a wooden bar attached to the bathroom wall, and with the doors removed from the hinges, Paul can move his wheelchair to the bathroom and can use the commode for elimination. Because of changes in his mobility pattern, and with no opportunity to walk, bowel habits are altered. Laxatives are now necessary and there are occasional accidents of soiled clothing because of difficulty in retaining loose feces. Urination is frequent due to the diuretic action of the hypertensive medication.

Comment

The distress that must accompany the difficulties with elimination is understandable. Paul is embarrassed when he soils his clothing. He is concerned and worried about the urinary frequency and his constant reflection and worry about elimination problems acts antagonistically to the blood pressure reducers. How can the cycle be interrupted? How can Paul be assured about the elimination alterations so that increased concern will not interfere with efforts to keep blood pressure stabilized? Is there any way to provide for physical activity that will promote more normal bowel elimination in particular? Is there sufficient motivation on Paul's part to pursue muscle strengthening activity to enable better muscle tone and better bowel elimination? Has he been instructed in muscle exercises?

Mobility

Rapid and hurried muscular activity were never part of Paul's life due to the palsy. With sufficient time allowed for movement about the home, the grounds outdoors, and for walking to friends' homes for visits, rather lengthy walks were taken regularly. From a physical standpoint, what is happening to the muscle tone now that movement is accomplished in the wheelchair? The leg and pelvic muscles employed for walking are being underutilized; the arm and shoulder muscles are being overutilized. Are muscles strengthening exercises being employed for shoulder and arm development? With what frequency and under what supervision? How effectively?

From a psychologic standpoint, what is Paul's reaction to wheelchair mobility? Does he enjoy it? Resent it? Is he depressed about being limited to the wheelchair? Does he enjoy the dependency on others? Is he engaging in muscle strengthening activity with the hope of becoming free of the wheelchair?

Communication

With a deaf person, communication requires specific skills and understanding. To interpret to Paul the pathology behind his palsy is just the beginning of the areas to explain to him—and probably the easiest area to be discussed. The most difficult areas to explain are the reasons for the hypertension, the numbness and tingling in his fingers and toes, the reasons for his decreased ability to walk, and the reasons for loss of fine coordination movements of the fingers. Medical diagnoses have been totally missing; causes have not been established.

Even if all these reasons were known, consider the variables in talking with a person who has been deaf all his life. What does "pain" mean to him? Can he differentiate "pain" from "ache"? "Dull' from "sharp"? "Intermittent" from "constant"? Does "numbness and tingling" mean the same to a deaf person as to a hearing person? Realizing that hearing persons, depending on their experiences and personalities, perceive these terms differently, consider the deaf person whose auditory input about pain has been appreciably less than that of a hearing person. The variables of experience and personality are there, too; but added variables of altered input compound the complexity of communication. Requirements for communication with Paul would include patience, adequate time to dialogue, facility with sign language and/or body language and/or pantomime.

One of the more difficult facets of communication is that of listening. At least, it seems that some persons have not mastered the art of listening. A deaf person, who is dependent for communication on his vision to observe lip movements, or to read written messages, or to interpret sign language and finger spelling, is probably more attentive to persons who are "speaking" to him than is the person who is able to hear. Intake of the spoken word can sometimes be separated in "hearing" and "listening." Sometimes a person hears words communicated to him but he may not always be listening to those words; his mind may be on other matters, or he may be threatened by invasion of his territory of knowledge. For example, Paul's family has been telling the physicians (general practitioners and psychiatrists) that Paul was "well" until six months ago. By "well," they are saying that Paul's health had not changed over the past 50 years. He is maintaining a level of wellness that is normal for him. The physicians have not been listening, apparently, because each of these medically educated persons has begun to instruct Paul's family about cerebral palsy—what it is, the types of palsy, etc. Paul's family is familiar with cerebral palsy, certainly not with the same medical orientation as the physicians, but with knowledge of the limitations of living as well as strengths of cerebral palsy victims. They are particularly aware of Paul's strengths and limitations, having lived and grown with him these 53 years.

How can one cope with the person who cannot listen? The patience, time, and sign language ability needed to cope with Paul's communication problems is different from the problem the family faces in dealing with the health professionals who do not listen. What language can the family use to communicate? How can the communication barriers between the family and the health personnel be removed, or at least reduced? These are major problems, not easy to resolve!

Summary Comment

Short range and long range goals need to be set for Paul, involving him in the goal-setting process as much as possible. Opportunity for frequent revision of goals is essential so that progress can be evaluated and obstacles to goal attainment identified. The ultimate goal is to return Paul to the level of functioning that existed prior to six months ago—to the range of function that was "normal" for him. Continued goals include:

1. Seeking motivators for Paul so that many of his activities will be self-initiated and self-maintained.
2. While making furniture arrangements, clothing placement, etc. to facilitate his independent movement, avoid encouraging dependency on others for everything.
3. Provide types of clothing that need limited buttoning, zipping, snapping, etc., so that fine finger movements are not necessary.
4. Set up a schedule of muscle activity to enhance muscle tone and muscle development, especially of the legs, hips, shoulders, and arms.
5. Arrange for periodic visits by those with whom Paul can communicate in order to promote feelings of self-worth and self-esteem. Permit conversation topics to be initiated by him. By doing this, certain clues about Paul's concerns or worries or needs might be elicited.
6. Periodically review with Paul the status of his pain as he perceives it, and observe carefully for unusual tension of facial features to indicate increasing pain, or altered body position to suggest increase in pain intensity.

Many other aspects of this multifaceted situation need to be explored. Extensive assessment has begun and needs to be continued, as is indicated by the questions raised in this overview of Paul's situation. The multidisciplinary approach and continued collaboration of many health team members and family members seems imperatve. Discouragement and frustration are "built-in" and inevitable in such a situation, but it is an excellent situation in which to use the nursing process. Identifying a few needs of the highest priority, then pursuing these through assessment, planning, implementing, and evaluating seems to be a reasonable approach. Each need, or group of needs, is looked on as a part of the total situation, and each is considered as an element in the adaptation to the continuation of these obvious deficits or removal of the deficits and a return to normalcy. Focusing on the activities of daily living is legitimate while setting goals to attain such functioning.

• *Situation: Ms. Bea Hardy at the Office of the Health Maintenance Organization (HMO)*

Ms. Bea Hardy is a successful professional person who has been actively engaged in business administrative activities since the age of 22. She has pursued further education while employed full time during all of these 25 years, and now, at the age of 47, at the peak of her career, is about to embark on something that is new to her. She is listening to a friend relate an experience of a health examination. Ms. Bea listens with more than the usual attention to her cohort's "check-up" experience. Should she, Ms. Bea, consider having the same examination? No, she thought; I have never been sick; why should I bother someone to request a "check-up" when I have no health problems? But then, she hesitated in thought—I am not getting any younger; maybe I should ask my friend for some more information about this service.

Ms. Bea's friend was most convincing in the narration of her experience. She told Ms. Bea about the lengthy questionnaire she filled out on entry to the office. The information they asked for was detailed and seemed to inquire about every facet of life; about her sleeping habits and pattern, eating habits, food preferences, tolerance for noise and for temperature—both heat and cold, her usual exercise and/or physical activity, her reaction to stress, ability to cope, and an extensive inquiry into her perceptions of herself as a person. With this introduction to her health examination experience, Ms. Bea's friend continued to share her very positive experience and she convinced Ms. Bea to arrange for her own health examination.

An appointment was made by Ms. Bea; she arrived at the HMO on the appointed day and was greeted by a nurse. The nurse reviewed the written health history that Ms. Bea had completed, and discussed several of the areas of the recorded data with Ms. Bea. From the conversation, the nurse was able to determine the gamut of tests that would be appropriate for her to have. Following the interview, the nurse asked Ms. Bea to disrobe and don a gown; then a thorough physical examination was done. Continued conversation with Ms. Bea during the examination elicited more data about her state of health.

While Ms. Bea was dressing after the examination, the nurse reviewed the data that had been collected via the interview, physical examination, and conversation; her analysis of the data led her to conclude that Ms. Bea demonstrated no apparent physical alteration and her psychologic state appeared to be within normal limits. Social and family histories suggested a stable pattern of living. Only one facet of the history raised some concern: there was a noticeable familial trait of diabetes in both parents, in the paternal grandparents, and in two paternal aunts. The nurse reviewed with the physician her concern about the diabetes potential and he agreed that a glucose tolerance test should be required along with the usual battery of tests. Together with Ms. Bea, the data were reviewed and they agreed that the only significant area elicited so far was the diabetes potential; further analysis would be done when the laboratory reports were received.

The necessary arrangements were made for Ms. Bea to return for the various X-Ray and laboratory tests. One week after her initial visit with the nurse, Ms. Bea returned, and all the test results were available. Analysis of the reports and a comparison with the assessment completed on the previous visit led the nurse and the doctor to the same conclusion: everything was within normal limits except the fasting blood sugar and the glucose tolerance test, these were borderline. With these data in hand, the nurse shared with Ms. Bea the findings of the examination and emphasized the diabetic potential. The need for maintenance of her present weight was stressed and Ms. Bea was urged to be alert to any weight gain. The nurse urged careful regulation of food intake to insure a balanced diet. A regular exercise program was recommended and it was suggested that some recreational and diversional activities should be interspersed with the professional activities.

To follow-up this initial health examination, Ms. Bea was advised to return to the HMO in one year for another examination; meanwhile, she should:

1. Conduct regular monthly breast self-examinations;
2. Walk at least one mile each day;

3. Maintain the intake of a balanced diet;
4. Control weight gain.

Although this was the first time that Ms. Bea had requested an examination to confirm her state of good health, it proved to be a positive experience, with good results.

Comment

As Americans become more knowledgeable about their health, they are assuming more responsibility for maintaining health. The availability of the nurse and the physician provided resources for Ms. Bea. These two health professionals combined their skills in assessing the strengths of Ms. Bea, assured her that she is in good health, identified a potential hazard that is evident but quiescent, and suggested adjustments in life style and habits to prevent the potential hazard from developing into an actual health problem. The conclusions reached as a result of the assessment were recorded and shared with Ms. Bea. In one year she will return to the HMO, where the assessment will be repeated, and the baseline data that were identified in this visit will be used to compare her status at that time.

Summary

The situations cited in this chapter are far from inclusive for all types of encounters that can confront nurses. The goal of these reports is to suggest the variety of age groups, settings, and problem areas the client may present. It will be necessary to devise different methods of coping with client problems, depending on the variables identified in each encounter. The orderly thought processes suggested in the four phases of the nursing process should make it easier for the nurse to cope with her responsibilities and assist the client to cope with his problems.

Chapter Five •

The Future of the Nursing Process

In the preceding chapters it was shown that the development and application of the nursing process provide evidence that this process is vital, ongoing, goal-directed, and logical. It is not only oriented to the present, but also to the future. This focus implies a continuum, linking the present to the future in a forward thrust.

The future of the nursing process cannot be predicted with certainty unless the events, trends, and changes of tomorrow are known. Speculations and predictions for mankind will have an impact on how, where, by whom, for whom, and when the nursing process will be utilized.

It may be well to ponder expectations for man in the future. The soaring sixties are a part of history, and recalling the events of the past can give direction to planning for the future. Change is now an accepted part of life, and it is safe to say that the only predictable certainty is the fact that change will occur. In future years, change will no doubt occur at an even faster pace than it has in the past.

When discussing change, it is important to think in terms of its rate and direction. For ". . . to define the content of change must include the consequences of pace itself. . . ."

Each person, whether a professional in the health field or a layman, can form a unique list of anticipated major health problems of the seventies. It seems clear that among the health problems in the United States are the following: (a) Pollution—air, water, land; contributing to this problem is that of overpopulation and the poor distribution of population. As more people occupy the earth, the amount of waste increases (liquid, solid, and gaseous). Crowding creates noise pollution; the metabolic processes of increasing numbers of people create more body waste, and increased food consumption creates more garbage. Each of these factors contributes to mental and physical health problems. (b) Drugs and alcohol —persons who take drugs, the care of persons who use drugs, and the reasons drugs and alcohol are used are of major concern. What makes a person, regardless of age, turn to drugs? Finding the answers to this question as well as coping with the problems created by the users is one of the major challenges of the late seventies.

The rising cost of health care is another of the major problems of the seventies. It is receiving much thought from many politicians, both candidates and elected officials. The debate about the involvement of the federal government contains vital issues to be resolved: the never-ending questions about the extent to which the federal government should or should not be involved in financing health care, the manner in which the state and federal governments should be responsible or share responsibility, and how they can do this without usurping the responsibility of local governments.

Continuing technical advancement without concomitant develment of, or the lagging development of, the philosophic, ethical, and moral implications of these advances are already presenting problems that may increase in the future. The impact of these developments on man and his environment, particularly those relating to genetic engineering, and designation of the time of death, are difficult questions to be answered; the term "sobering" may more accurately describe them. The prevention of illness continues to be emphasized as well as the curative and rehabilitative aspects of medicine.

How do these relate to the nursing process? These will be among the issues pertinent to nursing and necessary to the nursing process. For example, with emphasis on economics and on providing quality health care for the consumer of health services, a major issue will be the number of personnel needed, the kind of personnel, their training and education, their roles in health care, and their responsibilities. As more persons enter the area of nursing, can the consumer of nursing expect that having more nurses will mean receiving better care? Do nurses expect that the terms "more" and "better" can be equated?

The United States is a nation with some of the best medical resources in the world. Yet, its infant mortality rate is greater than that of at least ten other advanced countries. There are nations where only 5 percent of the national incomes goes to 20 percent of its families at the lowest end of the economic ladder, where malnutrition is a major problem, where care and inoculations are unknown. Rectifying these conditions is an ongoing challenge.[2]

Toffler suggests that future shock "may well be the most important disease of tomorrow." He defines future shock as ". . . a time phenomenon, a product of the greatly accelerated rate of change in society. . . . It is culture shock in one's society." It is his belief that man handles technologic innovation by going through the phases of idea creation, idea application, and idea diffusion.[1] To paraphrase Toffler and apply the steps to nursing, use of the nursing process would involve three phases:

1. There must be a creative, feasible idea and the suggestion that nursing can be of help in this situation; here is an area in which nursing offers some expertise to resolve or prevent a problem from developing.
2. The process must have a practical application. Having identified the area of need, assessed the problem or potential problem areas, and arrived at a plan for coping with them, the nurse must take some action. This action includes implementing as well as evaluating aspects of the process. Constant recycling through phases is an inherent part of the process.
3. The third phase in the utilization of the process involves "diffusion through society." Translated into the language of nursing, this involves convincing those who do nursing that orderly movement through the process insures the "how" of nursing; it insures the systematic and orderly movement through necessary phases of nursing so that problems of clients can be thoroughly assessed, action for coping can be planned and implemented, and a final and continual evaluation becomes as essential as is each of the other three phases of the process.

Thus, challenges for the future of society, of health care, and of nursing care are coming into focus. The nursing process will significantly meet some of these challenges.

The future of the nursing process is seen from four points of view:

1. Continuing development and refinement of the process itself,
2. Contribution toward the growth and development of the profession of nursing through its use,
3. Influences on the personal and professional growth and the development of users of the nursing process, and
4. Improvement of the health status of recipients of the process.

Deliberate use of the nursing process by nursing practitioners will contribute to the refinement of its component elements. Improved history taking, more accurate nursing diagnoses, more effective priority setting, improved design of nursing care plans, more astute specifications of expected client behaviors, more effective recording of observations about the client, more sensible, purposeful and effective nurse actions, more emphasis on evaluation as well as on the development of tools for evaluation, and better judgment concerning what to communicate to whom, and when to communicate and how, are goals of the continuing development of the nursing process.

Numerous authors have developed tools and techniques that are incorporated into the nursing process. Continuing development, testing, and refinement of these tools in a variety of health care settings with the nurse and other nursing and health team members are in order. Formulating a theoretical base for shortening the time lag between the discovery of a new method, or of new knowledge, and its incorporation into nursing practice deserves serious attention in the formulation of a full framework for applying the nursing process.

The contribution of the nursing process to growth and development of the profession of nursing is easily evidenced. Because the heart of the nursing practice is the designation and solution of client problems, any theories or scientific materials developed to explain, direct, or influence nursing practice will contribute to the quality of service rendered the client and hence advance the profession and sanction its place as designated by society. A case in point would be the study and analysis of the content of nursing care plans. In Chapter 3, it was recommended that nursing care plans be developed in their entirety and retained for future study and analysis. Well-designed and complete nursing care plans would contribute a wealth of data about a client, his problems, solutions to those problems, and the effectiveness of these solutions. Research is inherent in the process. Hunches, observations, and speculations lend themselves to further research and testing. Nursing care plans can be analyzed according to many variables—age, sex, educational level, level of wellness, level of illness, common problems, unique problems, solutions and their effectiveness, the predictable level of success from alternative solutions, and determining the status of solutions. The careful, analytical extraction and testing of data will contribute to the development of nursing theory. Nursing care plans, nursing histories, and associated observations and results can be used to develop model care plans for males and females in a particular setting, of a particular age, with a particular problem, having certain resources. These models can enhance the nurse's role as a client specialist.

When considering the influence of the nursing process on the nurse's personal and professional growth and development, as a person and as a practitioner, a few topics need to be considered. For example, the nursing process as a process and functional entity should be a major component of continuing education, which would include its present use as well as additional areas for use in a practice setting. The problem-solving that results from the nursing process is a fruitful area, replete with a multitude of situations that could be shared with colleagues for their enlightenment and reaction.

The nursing process lends itself to the nurse's own quest for self-improvement. Continuous evaluation of one's intellectual, interpersonal, and technical skills and one's perceptual, communicative, and decision-making ability will reveal strengths and limitations. Interest in enhancing one's strengths and minimizing one's limitations gives direction for study and the selection of programs, workshops, and professional associations and interactions. Improvement in areas of history-taking, nursing diagnoses, and listening, to mention a few, can be a lifelong endeavor. Increasing one's accuracy in problem-solving and in predicting the impact on client behavior are important factors in experiencing success in nursing practice. The continuing focus on self-improvement results in the better use of self and improved contribution to citizens. The nursing process, therefore, can be viewed as an effective method to prevent and minimize obsolescence.

The client will benefit most from a nurse who is knowledgeable, confident, creative, and person-centered. Whether his situation demands that wellness be maintained, care be given during acute or chronic illness, or compassionate support rendered if he is dying, he will be the recipient of the best care the nurse has to offer. The nurse, too, will be stimulated to continue her self-development, as she reaps the feeling of accomplishment from giving her best. Inherent in this feeling of success is a realistic appraisal of oneself and the client situation. It involves being able to accept a setback without being unduly crushed, being able to strive forward despite odds, and being convinced that one's contribution is the best that can be given at a particular time.

The client further benefits by active participation in the identification and resolution of his problems. It enhances his personhood, his need to remain a thinking, feeling person whether he is well or ill, and his need to maximize the well portion of his being although he is afflicted by some disability.

The nursing process contributes to the nurse's feeling of camaraderie with other members of the health team. She values her contributions and enhances the success of the health professionals by sharing her perceptions and goals for the client. Her success is, in turn, enhanced by her being open and receptive to suggestions of nursing and health team members.

Inherent in each deliberation of the future of the nursing process is the research process. Presently, the need for clinical research is generally recognized by nurse practitioners, and the quantity and quality of clinical nursing research will predictably improve in the next decade. The need for increased research in nursing practice is documented in *Abstract for Action,* a report of the National Commission for the Study of Nursing and Nursing Education. The report clearly demonstrates the need for a body of facts and a set of probabilities to guide or assess the nursing care of citizens. A clear knowledge of the differences in the benefits to the client from nursing interventions and establishment of means to assess the results of varied interventions are based on sound research.[3]

Research plays an important role in the development and refinement of the nursing process and in the development of nursing science. Sharing the results of research can benefit the nurse and the client directly. The nursing process opens the way for research not only into a multitude of problems but also into each component with each of its elements, which is itself a fruitful area for research. Fox developed a useful model for identifying research problems in nursing. The model is based on the nursing process and includes numerous helpful suggestions for research by nurses alone or by nurses in collaboration with other health professionals. To summarize the suggestions of Fox,[4] the following types of research studies may be undertaken:

1. Those related to health needs, health personnel consulted about health needs and the medical and nursing care plan.
2. Those related to decisions inherent in the nursing process.
3. Those related to the professional role and the legal limit of the practice of nursing.
4. Those related to the setting in which the nursing process is utilized.
5. Those related to the utilization of the nursing process by nurses with varying backgrounds in education and experience.
6. Those related to the roles of the client, his family, and other professional and nonprofessional personnel in implementing the nursing care plan.
7. Those relating to the impact of direct nursing care on the client, and
9. Those relating to the communication of data.[4]

Specifically, any of the following studies, as well as a multitude of others, can be undertaken with the hope that the results would contribute to the continuing development of the nursing process, comprise a nursing science, and contribute to an increase in the caliber of care rendered to citizens:

1. Comparative studies of nursing histories taken by nurses with differing educational and practice backgrounds and functioning in a variety of settings.
2. Studies of the utilization of the nursing history and health assessment in the development of the nursing care plan.
3. Studies of the client's reaction to self-completion of the nursing history form, with and without personal interview.
4. Studies of the number and kind of decisions made based on data of the nursing history and health assessment for well and ill clients.
5. Comparative studies of the number and kinds of decisions made by nurses in varying settings and with different backgrounds of education and experience.
6. Studies of whether a selected number of nurses, given the same set of data, would make the same nursing diagnoses. If there is variation, studies of this variation according to education, experience, and culture of the nurses.
7. Studies to determine why the nurse selects a particular strategy or action for a client based on a selected nursing diagnosis and the client variables considered in making the selection.

8. Studies of what constitutes the data base to support the making of a nursing diagnosis for the client. Comparative studies could be done contrasting the data base and nursing diagnosis(es) made by nurses with the baccalaureate, the masters, and the doctoral degrees *in nursing*.
9. Studies of how different citizens with a similar health problem resolve this problem.
10. Studies of varying patterns of problem resolution according to age, sex, geographic location, socioeconomic level, and educational and cultural background.
11. Studies to analyze the first encounter of the nurse and client in terms of why the client sought out the nurse. Studies to determine if the nurse was the first member of the health team to enter the client into the health care system or if the encounter resulted from his prior interaction with a physician or other health team member.
12. Studies to define the client's role in the development of the nursing care plan.
13. Studies to determine factors that comprise the rationale for setting priorities for client problems. A study of whether this priority setting is aected by differences in the nurse's education and experience and those of the client. Comparative studies of priority setting for client problems, as designated by the nurse and the client. If there is a conflict in priority setting, a study of the factors inherent in the conflict.
14. When eliciting solutions to client problems, studies should be done to determine how to recognize the best solution.
15. Studies to determine factors inherent in the nurse's decision to refer or not refer a client problem to another health care professional or another agency.
16. Studies of perceptions and observations about the client that are recorded and shared in contrast to those withheld. Analytical studies of the data withheld and the rationale for withholding them. Studies of the nurse's education and experience in contrast to the quantity and quality of data withheld.
17. Studies to determine variations of and common solutions made by nurses in different settings when confronted with a given client problem, a designated number of staff, and selected equipment and supplies.
18. A study of the rationale for delegating actions to be performed by members of the nursing team rather than by the nurse herself.

19. Studies of the impact of agency policies on the number, kinds, and quality of decisions made by the nurse relative to assessing, planning, implementing, and evaluating care.
20. Studies to develop tools to evaluate the impact of nurse actions on client behavior.
21. Studies to determine the client's role in evaluating the nursing care rendered to him.
22. Studies of the impact of the client's evaluation on subsequent nurse actions designated to solve problems.
23. Studies of how effectively nurses evaluate nursing care.
24. Studies to determine the extent to which nurses transfer or reproduce decisions utilized in one situation to another.
25. Studies of inherent factors in a situation that foster or deter the transfer or reproduction of decisions.
26. Studies to determine why, when, what, and how nurses use research findings and incorporate them into their use of the nursing process.

In addition to the recommended nursing research studies, it is imperative that nurses use the research findings related to human behavior and incorporate these into nursing practice.

Experiences in nursing have suggested two subject areas that particularly warrant exploration—periodicity and territoriality. The limited data already obtained from applications of these two concepts to nursing suggest that there is a vast and rich potential that will contribute qualitatively to improved nursing and client care.

Periodicity is the cycle through which all living matter moves; the cycle is characterized by a regular pattern of peaks and troughs. Periodicity is also known as biologic rhythm, circadian rhythm, body rhythm, body clock, and by a variety of other labels. The cyclic nature of the physical environment is discernible in the changing seasons of the year, in the change from day to night, in the blossoming of flowers and their return to seed, and in the annual harvesting of fields. The cyclic nature of the human body is evident by mood swings that people experience on a daily, monthly, or seasonal basis, by daily and monthly fluctuations in body weight, by the increase and decrease in appetite on a cyclic basis, by the sleep-wake cycle, and by many other parameters.

The advent of space travel has accelerated the need for understanding the time adjustment of the body clocks. Intercontinental travel by jet planes provides speedy movement across datelines, yet it has become necessary to plan time schedules to allow body clocks to adjust to the change. For example, businessmen who travel to

Paris must allow a 24- to 48-hour period for body systems to synchronize with the surrounding environment to provide for optimum functioning.

When one attempts to apply this concept of periodicity to client care, a number of questions are raised. To what extent is the client's body clock considered when planning for medication administration? Studies show that people are more susceptible to medication effects at certain times of the 24-hour period than at other times of the day. The peaks and troughs of metabolic activity account for this difference in receptivity to medication intake. Can nurses contribute to the collection of data that will provide a profile of client periodicity patterns? Are there certain times of the day when clients may be more mentally alert, more receptive to instructions about health and nursing care, about rehabilitation measures, about taking medications at home?

These are some of the many questions one can raise relating to the concept of periodicity. Although time and study will be necessary to provide more complete data, the work should be initiated. Gradual but sure inroads into such concepts will be highly beneficial to the client and to the nurse.

The concept of territoriality (a relatively new one in the natural and behavioral sciences) applies to that area of space (earth, air, or water) a person defines and defends as his own. Studies show that animate beings possess an inner compulsion to own their own territory and exert a marked effort to defend it. Some authors see the territorial nature of man as a genetic trait that cannot be eradicated.[5] If one accepts this inherent quality in man, a number of questions can be raised relative to the territorial rights of clients with whom nurses function.

How does the client's territory concern the nurse? When a nurse enters a client's home, it is not difficult to identify territorial rights and respect them. When a client comes to a clinic, a hospital, or other agency to seek help from health personnel, his territory grows smaller but does not vanish. It becomes a more circumscribed area of smaller dimensions surrounding his person. In the hospital, the client's territory is usually limited to the area surrounding the bed, including the bedside table, the chair, and the bed itself. Clients usually refer to the lack of privacy in the hospital as a violation of personal space rather than an invasion of territory.[6] A certain amount of intrusion of personal space by personnel is necessary and expected when a person becomes ill. An awareness of the client's personal space is important to his care and the nurse must be concerned with his reaction to her intrusion. Responses to actions of others can change as one becomes ill. An event to which one would not react when healthy may create a marked reaction when ill. An intrusion or invasion of one's space or territory can represent a threat to the ill person. The reaction to the threat is essentially one in which the inherent drive to defend one's property is activated. The nurse must think of this mechanism when she is observing the client's behavior and assessing his situation.

A study by Crenshaw revealed 45 incidents in which 30 patients described what they perceived as unnecessary invasions of privacy. She assumed that invasion of privacy is one manifestation of the invasion of personal space. More than half of the invasions were by nursing personnel, most of whom were professional nurses.[7]

Although the disciplines of anthropology, sociology, and psychology have studied this concept of space and territory, nursing has made only minor inroads into this subject. However, the fascinating potential of exploring this concept to determine its possible application to nursing should prove very exciting to practicing nurses. Those with pioneer spirits will find much data on which to build some "hunches," suggest some hypotheses, and explore realistically, in some depth, when helping clients in a variety of settings. Fertile areas for discovery can stimulate more growth and development in the nursing profession than has yet been realized. The major requirements are a willing mind and enthusiasm for the continued improvement of self and service to others.

Thus, the nursing process can give rise to areas for nursing research, and the tools and data realized through the deliberate use of the nursing process can provide data for that research.

The quality of the nursing process in the practice of nursing and its involvement in research in nursing practice will be the basis for the certification of nurse specialists. This recognition for members of the profession by the membership will designate a high level of quality in service rendered to citizens. Among means to be utilized as evidence to support claims of excellence are written descriptions of problem-solving or the use of the nursing process in a selection of nurse–client encounters. These descriptions will be subject to peer review. The evaluation inherent in the process itself, followed by an evaluation by peers incorporating standards of practice, supports the conviction that nurse practitioners have accepted the fact that they are accountable for these actions. While nursing has already agreed to accept this responsibility, citizen demand that health care personnel, political leaders, lawyers, and businessmen, to mention a few, be accountable for their actions will be increased and strengthened during the coming decade.

Accountability suggests responsibility, an obligation to answer to someone. Legally, a nurse can be held accountable for her actions as well as her inactions. Implicit within this obligation is the suggestion that the nurse is expected to have certain basic knowledge; she is obliged to make decisions, and to use judgment based on that knowledge. Within this context she is responsible for taking appropriate actions, whether interdependent or independent.

Implementation of independent actions by the nurse requires careful adherence to the nursing process to determine the scope of her responsibility and to insure fulfillment of the kind of actions necessary to help the client. As interdependent actions are necessary, the nurse visualizes responsibilities along several avenues; she continually keeps in mind her responsibility to the client and his family, yet simultaneously is aware of her accountability to herself, to other nursing and health team members, and to her employer, if she is not an independent practitioner. Hence, this mosaic of accountability and responsibility takes on many dimensions. As these facets continually present themselves to the nurse practitioner, she is accountable for taking some action. If no action is taken when one is necessary, or when a legal action can prove a nursing action should have been taken, then the nurse is accountable. Thus, future responsibility is inherent in all present acts.

The primary focus for the nurse is the client and his problems. For helping the client to cope with actual or potential health needs, the nurse is directly accountable to him. Because the client is always viewed as an integral part of a family unit, the nurse is accountable to the client's family, in either a primary or a secondary way, or in a direct or indirect way.

Of particular significance in the nurse's accountability is the need to operationalize, in nursing practice, the belief that man is a unique, holistic being. The nursing client reflects the multicultural society with its religious, economic, geographic, ethnic, racial, and cultural heritage and dimensions. The nurse must be sensitive to and account for the role of this heritage and these dimensions when rendering nursing service to the client. In this era of renewed cultural, ethnic, geographic, racial, and religious sensitivity, it is strategic that the nurse refrain from creating minority groups among clients by overvaluing or undervaluing any or all of these human dimensions. Minorities are created, not born. It is nursing's responsibility, first and foremost, to render health and nursing care to *all* persons. The nursing process requires that *full* data about persons and families be sought in order to assess, plan, implement and evaluate nursing services rendered.

Through the use of the nursing process quality care is rendered for all persons and families with full consideration of age, sex, creed, ethnic origin, race, life style, occupation, and geographic location. Failure to consider these dimensions in nursing care results in haphazard, depersonalized, and ineffective care—the basis for causing problems rather than solving health care problems.

Exclusive attention of the nurse to one selected variable or dimension of the person such as sex, ethnic origin, creed, or race results in a failure to render complete care and, therefore, demonstrates that the nurse does not recognize nor appreciate the wholeness of man. Nursing's responsibility is to the maintenance of the integrity of the basic human needs of people.

Only when nursing fails to fulfill its commitment to all people rather than to one aspect of cultural diversity or economic status are minorities produced. Minorities are the result of society's and nursing's failure to support and implement a belief in the dignity of all persons and also a result of a failure to utilize the nursing process appropriately to render nursing care to clients and their families. Nursing's responsibility is to operationalize beliefs in man's rights, roles, relationships, and diversity; to help develop an environment in which persons can maintain their well-being individually and in collaboration with others; to support man's striving and achieving optimal wellness, and to assist and to facilitate this accomplishment. Thus, the nursing process is a viable safeguard and the best protection for holistic, dignified, effective nursing service.

Every nurse is accountable to herself. She knows best her intentions and she can best explain to what extent she is accountable. Usually, if the nurse is comfortably sure that she has measured up to the demands of accountability to herself, then her accountability to others can be successful.

Accountability for solving the client's problems is shared by all members of nursing and health teams. A liaison exists because of their mutual concern, the welfare of the client. In addition, a collaborative and an ethical role exists among personnel. The nurse is primarily responsible for instrumental functions of group cohesion as well as for the expressive functions of moving the group toward defined goals.

Another facet of accountability and responsibility is the willingness to share experiences through the professional publication of practical experiences. The nurse involved in using the nursing process will accumulate qualitative and quantitative physiologic and behavioral data about a client, which are available to few persons. The critical analysis of these data will render valuable information to serve as guidelines for the nurse's future actions. The data provide benefits for herself; in addition the nurse has a professional responsibility to share them with her colleagues, not only to enlighten them, but to stimulate their thinking and to propose ideas to a forum for reaction, refinement, and development by other members of the nursing profession. This sharing fosters the growth and development of the profession. The personal accumulation of valuable data benefits only one or two persons. Sharing this information with one's colleagues extends its value many fold. Not only will the value of the data be made known, but weaknesses and inaccuracies will be pointed out in an objective way, which, in turn, should benefit the sharer of that information. Solutions to problems, reactions of clients to solutions, the development of techniques and procedures, the recognition of problems unique and common to a person and/or setting, would serve as the basis for professional writing. Publishing the results of research by nurse practitioners gives the reader a basis for making judgments about the results and also gives her some knowledge of the research that has been completed, eliminating duplication. The published research study can serve as a model for future research.

Participating and writing in conjunction with other members of the health team can foster relationships and mutual understanding of each contributor's point of view and role. This health team and interdisciplinary collaboration is strategic in those settings and with those client problems that involve combined input from the nurse, the physician, the dentist, the clinical pharmacist, the social worker, and so on.

In addition to its future role in research, the nursing process will play a significant part in fulfilling resolutions passed by the members of the National League for Nursing and the American Nurses Association which have an impact on the future health care of citizens. Selectively, resolutions urge a speedy passage of health legislation that would make high quality health care readily accessible to all segments of society. All aspects of health care services should be available, with greater emphasis on preventive as well as therapeutic aspects and with special attention to financing mechanisms and appropriate cost control. It was resolved that a conference on health care be held to discuss the full range of preventive services, manpower needs, facilities, financing, and distribution of services.

Emphasis on the use of home health services should be continued and action initiated and maintained to avoid duplication of such services at the community level. Existing home health care agencies presently providing client care should be used in any community level development, restructuring, or reorganization of health care services.

One resolution supported the identification of nomenclature and development of a classification system for nursing diagnoses. Another included a statement that skilled nursing is a composite of on-going observation, judgment, management, counseling, teaching, and direct care as well as the implementation of a nursing care plan in conjunction with the medical care plan.

The nursing care plan must be evaluated and revised as indicated, and the client's needs and responses must be documented. Inherent in this resolution is national sanction for the nursing process. Still another resolution stated that nursing shares responsibility for the health and welfare of the community and of the individual with health problems. A resolution was also passed, reaffirming preventive nursing care to the family as a unit and, in the event the client dies, support for the continuing services needed by the family.

Resolutions and position papers have been developed in support of the direct access to nursing service by the client and direct payment by private and public third party payers to qualified nurses for nursing care rendered to clients and their families. Implicit in this request is the *just* remuneration for these services. Direct payment to qualified nurses is long overdue. Mastery of the use of the nursing process should be the basis for fair payment for nursing services rendered. The nursing process can provide the framework for designation of costs and fees, cost effective accounting, and for overall accountability for nursing services provided.

Other resolutions reaffirmed the commitment to care for and serve as advocate for the aged and terminally ill clients, to improve the care and services to the elderly, and to participate actively with health care professionals and parents in planning and meeting the needs of mothers and children. Significantly, a resolution has been passed to exercise the *Code for Nurses* and to provide a mechanism for reporting and handling incompetent, unethical, or illegal practice. This resolution supports the emphasis placed on the profession's accountability for its product or practice. The nursing process, with its built-in evaluation, would be the effective means for implementing this accountability.

It was resolved that peer review be provided in every health care facility to maintain standards of care. Implicit in this resolution is support for high-quality nursing practice for the citizen and the professional maturity that comes with the willingness to accept responsibility for one's acts and a desire to subject them to the scrutiny of one's peers. What better way is there to supply evidence that the nursing process has been used than by nursing histories and health assessments, nursing diagnoses, nursing orders, nursing care plans and their revisions and/or modifications? Another resolution stated that the Congress for Nursing and the divisions of practice develop mechanisms whereby clinical specialists define their role, qualifications, and responsibilities in nursing practice.

Learning programs in both the basic and continuing education programs were called on to provide learning opportunities for competence in primary health care practice. The nursing process can be used effectively by the nurse engaged in primary health care. Continued education received considerable emphasis. The nursing process affords an almost endless number of topics and directions that can be pursued for inservice and continuing education purposes based on data obtained about clients, their problems, and solutions.

Many other resolutions have been passed—all directly or indirectly geared to improve health services to the citizen. Some urged that all billing and reimbursement procedures clearly identify the nature and cost of nursing services. Others related to the need for effective health legislation to assure the needed health manpower. Inherent in the nursing manpower needs is strong support for the preparation of nurses at the masters and doctoral levels in nursing as specialist nursing practitioners, teachers and administrators of nursing, consultants, and researchers. A nationwide moratorium on licensing additional health occupations was supported, as were sound licensing laws. The commitment to individual accountability and individual licensure as essential to high quality safe care was strongly reaffirmed. All resolutions will have an implication for the immediate and distant future. The nursing process as a process and its outcomes are strategic to fulfill these client-centered resolutions.

Results of the study of nursing and nursing education by the National Commission for the Study of Nursing and Nursing Education broadly outline the need to increase clinical nursing research and research related to nurse education. It confirms the need to clarify roles and practices in conjunction with other health professions to ensure the delivery of optimum health care and the need for increased financial support for nurses and nursing so that appropriate numbers and types of nurses are prepared to meet present and future demands for quality health care in the years to come.[3]

Considering the resolutions and recommendations that point to the future focus for nurses and nursing, it appears that nurses will be intellectually, interpersonally, and technically busy. The nursing process, as the key to quality nursing practice, will be an important part of future nursing practice.

To conclude our presentation on the nursing process, we would like to repeat this often-quoted story: A chicken and a pig were walking down the street. As they walked they came to a billboard displaying a breakfast of ham and eggs. The chicken said to the pig, "Look at the wonderful contribution I have made to mankind." The pig listened, then said, "Yes, that's fine, but my contribution involves a total commitment!"

References

1. Toffler A: Future Shock, part 1. New York, Random House, 1970, pp 1–50
2. The stormy 70's—big changes still to come. Changing Times 26:25–31, 1972
3. Lysaught J: An Abstract for Action. New York, McGraw-Hill, 1970, pp 84–155
4. Fox DJ: Fundamentals of Research in Nursing, 3rd edition. New York, Appleton-Century-Crofts, 1976, pp 61–66
5. Ardrey R: The Territorial Imperative. New York, Atheneum, 1966, pp 1–155
6. Sommer R, Dewar R: The physical environment of the ward. Freidson E (ed): The Hospital in Modern Society. New York, Free Press of Glencoe, 1963
7. Crenshaw AE: Invasion of Personal Space as Perceived by a Selected Group of Patients. Unpublished Masters Dissertation, School of Nursing, The Catholic University of America, Washington DC, May 1972

Appendices •

• *Appendix A*
National and International Codes for Nurses

The Code for Nurses (National)

1. The nurse provides services with respect for human dignity and the uniqueness of the client unrestricted by considerations of social or economic status, personal attributes, or the nature of the health problems.
2. The nurse safeguards the client's right to privacy by judiciously protecting information of a confidential nature.
3. The nurse acts to safeguard the client and the public when health care and safety are affected by the incompetent, unethical, or illegal practice of any person.
4. The nurse assumes responsibility and accountability for individual nursing judgments and actions.
5. The nurse maintains competence in nursing.
6. The nurse exercises informed judgment and uses individual competence and qualifications as criteria in seeking consultation, accepting responsibilities, and delegating nursing activities to others.
7. The nurse participates in activities that contribute to the ongoing development of the profession's body of knowledge.
8. The nurse participates in the profession's efforts to establish, implement and improve standards of nursing.
9. The nurse participates in the profession's efforts to establish and maintain conditions of employment conducive to high quality nursing care.
10. The nurse participates in the profession's effort to protect the public from misinformation and misrepresentation and to maintain the integrity of nursing.
11. The nurse collaborates with members of the health professions and other citizens in promoting community and national efforts to meet the health needs of the public.

Code for Nurses. Am Nurse 8(14):5, October 15, 1976.

The Code for Nurses (International)

The fundamental responsibility of the nurse is fourfold: to promote health, to prevent illness, to restore health and to alleviate suffering.

The need for nursing is universal. Inherent in nursing is respect for life, dignity and rights of man. It is unrestricted by considerations of nationality, race, creed, color, age, sex, politics or social status.

Nurses render health services to the individual, the family and the community and coordinate their services with those of related groups.

Nurses and People. The nurse's primary responsibility is to those people who require nursing care. The nurse, in providing care, respects the beliefs, values, and customs of the individual. The nurse holds in confidence personal information and uses judgment in sharing this information.

Nurses and Practice. The nurse carries personal responsibility for nursing practice and for maintaining competence by continual learning. The nurse maintains the highest standards of nursing care possible within the reality of a specific situation. The nurse uses judgment in relation to individual competence when accepting and delegating responsibilities. The nurse, when acting in a professional capacity, should at all times maintain standards of personal conduct that would reflect credit on the profession.

Nurses and Society. The nurse shares with other citizens the responsibility for initiating and supporting action to meet the health and social needs of the public.

Nurses and Co-workers. The nurse sustains a cooperative relationship with co-workers in nursing and other fields. The nurse takes appropriate action to safeguard the individual when his care is endangered by a co-worker or any other person.

Nurses and the Profession. The nurse plays the major role in determining and implementing desirable standards of nursing practice and nursing education. The nurse is active in developing a core of professional knowledge. The nurse, acting through the professional organization, participates in establishing and maintaining equitable social and economic working conditions in nursing.

1973 Code for Nurses. Am J Nurs 73:1351, August 1973.

• *Appendix B*
Selected Observations Made Using Four Senses

The following is a list of observations that can be made by the nurse through the use of her four senses—seeing, hearing, smelling, and touching.

I. Observations Made by Seeing

  a. The Client

    1. General appearance and visible mood expression. Male, female, infant, child, adolescent, young adult, middle-aged adult, older adult, aged, estimation of age, age appropriateness, younger-appearing, older-appearing, clean, unkempt, tall, slim, short, malnourished, obese, plump, wasting, lean, emaciated, well-nourished, gigantism, dwarfism, thin, sad, happy, bored, anxious, fearful, eager, alert, flat affect, Down's syndrome, hostile, suspicious, attentive, sleepy, staring, tearful, frowning, inattentive, nervous, depressed, hyperactive, hyperalert, conscious, preoccupied, distressed, jittery, crying, disoriented, clowning, comatose, unconscious, nonresponsive, stuporous, weak, shaking chill, appearing ill
    2. Visible physical factors
      a. Head and neck area: macrocephalic, microcephalic, normocephalic, goiter, tumors, swelling, infections, tics, fontanels-bulging, pulsating, closed; paralysis, stiffness, congenital malformations, scars, hematoma, moonface, mask of pregnancy
      b. Hair: amount, distribution—male, female, adult, child, normal, sparse, unusual hairiness, complete baldness, bald spots; texture—fine, coarse, brittle, split ends; color—natural, dyed; baldness—scattered, circumscribed, extensive; long, short, straight, braided, curled, coiffured, bearded, mustache, simply combed, unkempt, oily, lice, ringworm, hair cosmetics and jewelry, hairpieces, wigs, dandruff
      c. Eyes: strabismus, tearing, swollen lids, stye, ecchymotic, conjunctiva-shiny, red, moist, smooth, clear, reddened, irritated; restricted or uneven eye movements; eye makeup, shaggy eyebrows, tweezed eyebrows, ptosis of lids—symmetrical, unequal; bulging eyes, slanted

eyes, squinting eyes, puffy lids, photophobic eyes, cataracts, blinking, eyeglasses–regular, bifocals, trifocals, sunglasses, reading, tinted, light sensitive; contact lenses, artificial eyes; pupils–regular, irregular, dilated, contracted; blind, twitching, sleeping, squinting

d. Nose: small, pugnosed, enlarged, distorted, draining-mucus, blood, purulent; normal septum, septal deviation; tumors, dilated nares, pinched nares, scabs, crusts, foreign objects

e. Ears: normal, enlarged, small, absent, deformed–congenital, cauliflower; drainage–bloody, purulent, crusting, clotting, waxy; tympanic membrane-glistening, pearly, red, inflamed, ruptured; swelling in front of and/or behind, foreign objects, jewelry-pierced ears, earrings

f. Lips, mouth and teeth: tongue-smooth, hairy, ulcerated, protruding, tongue-tie, swollen, coated, distorted, lacerated, excised, lesion, short frenulum; lips–moist, parched, fiery red, cracked, lipstick, presence of food, gum, tobacco, toys in mouth; dentures–partial, full; teeth-full dentition; primary, secondary, protruding, missing replaced, missing unreplaced, transplanted, capped, crowned, broken, gold inlay, decayed, loose; stained teeth–tea, coffee, tobacco, drugs; fillings–minimal, copious, crowns, caps, gold; hairlip, cleft palate–repaired, unrepaired, twitching, scars, distorted configuration, malocclusion, chancre, vomiting –projectile; air swallowing, mouth breathing, normal breathing, difficult breathing, drooling; herpes simplex, tumors, swelling, paralysis, lipstick, eating, vomiting, sucking, drinking, yawning, sneezing, sordes, teeth chattering, postnasal drip

g. Skin: Clear, full, firm, plump, thin, aged, warm, cold, dirty, crusted, blushing, bruised, cuts, scratches, abrasions, fistulae, ecchymoses, sinuses; elevations–tumors, warts, blisters, boils, carbuncles, abscesses, pimples, pustules, hives, pox, papules; chafed, sunburn, burns, flaking, distribution of fat in and under the skin, facial butterfly lesion, gangrene, necrosis, petechiae, cracks, fissures, peeling, scaly, rashes–circumscribed, profuse, generalized; acne, hemorrhage, scars, keloid, punctures, vaccination scar, venipuncture, venipuncture scars; color–racial, nationality, hereditary–redhead, blonde, brunette, brown, black; pathologic color —jaundice, pallor, too rosy, cyanotic, mottling; goose flesh; infestation—pin worms, lice; drainage—serous, serosanguinous, bloody, mucus, purulent; callouses, corns, bunions, tattoos, hairy, absence of hair, protrusion of veins, network of nestlike veins, attached umbilical cord, healed umbilicus, sweaty, dehydrated; soiled—urine, blood, feces, purulent material, dirt, other substances such as tar, adhesive marks, discolored—gentian violet, potassium permanganate, silver nitrate, tincture of benzoin; presence of powders, pastes, deodorants, jewelry, tumor, hernia, decubiti, ulcers, radiation markings, sutures, diaper rash, prickly heat, nails—well groomed, bitten, hangnails, ridges, grooves, absence of nailpolish, artificial, pitting

h. Posture: position; erect, upright, straight without support, unsteady, straight with support—braces, cane, crutches, walker; distorted—kyphosis, lordosis, scoliosis, shoulders curved, stooped, wry neck, wrenched; pacing, rigid, shuffling gait, foot dragging, lame, sitting-legs and feet relaxed, knees crossed, ankles crossed, swinging legs, in chair, on floor, painful, unable to get up from chair or floor, in wheelchair, on edge of bed; dorsal recumbent, side lying, supine, prone, jackknife, opisthotonos, Fowler's, semi-Fowler's, dorsal lithotomy, knee-chest, immobile, mobile; walking—slowing, rapidly, limping, shivering, awkward, kneeling, squatting, jumping, creeping, crawling, running, fainting, sleep walking, convulsing, writhing, unusual position, palsied, shaking chills, stiffness posture of late pregnancy, sleeping soundly, restless; sidelying position, fetal position, immersed in bedclothes, uncovered, supine, still, prone

i. Extremities: Extended, paralyzed, flaccid, spastic; absence of portion (fingers, toes) or all of extremity, contractures, clubbing of fingers and toes, foot drop, hand drop, artificial limb, mongoloid palm, asymmetry, extragluteal fold, wringing hands, tapping feet, kicking, edematous, discolored, crippled, clubfoot, knockknees, varicosities, red and inflamed, hairy; stained extremities—occupational dyes, tar, nicotine; fingernails and toenails—short, manicured, long, dirty, bitten, hangnails, blood blister, cracked, chipped, ridged, pitted, absent; arch supports, corrective shoes, bunions, barefeet, unequal limb length, bow legs, excessive muscle development, minimal muscle development, fissures and cracks between toes and fingers, dislocation, fractures—green stick, compound; gangrene, parts cut out of shoes, bandages, bandaids, clenched fist, clutching items, clean hands and feet, soiled hands—dirt, blood, body secretions; tremors, trembling, swelling, weak reflexes, exaggerated reflexes, twitching, flapping, picking, pushing, holding, clapping, patting, scratching, touching, frostbitten, left-handed, right-handed, ambidextrous, handshake—firm grip, tense, anxious, loose, too hard, weak, cold, sweating, limp, flaccid, fleeting, hot dry, calloused, unusually soft.

j. Trunk area: breathing—rhythmic, arrhythmic, breathholding, absence of; barrel chest, protruding ribs, absence of rib, scars, tumors, burns, abrasions, lacerations, pulsations, swelling, distortions, fat distribution, discolorations; breasts—developing, mature, child, male, female, enlarged, symmetric, asymmetric, lactating; nipples—normal nonparous, parous, cracked, inverted, bleeding, absence of breast; silicone implantation, surgical alterations; colostomy; gastrostomy, ileostomy; abdomen-flat, protruding, distended, obese, pregnant; scars, striae; back-spina bifida, pilonidal sinus; hemorrhage, incisions; puncture; hernia-umbilical, inguinal, incisional, fetal movements in late pregnancy, intestinal movement, obvious organ enlargement—liver, spleen

k. Pelvic and genital area: male, female, infant, child, adolescent, adult, congenital anomalies, surgical alterations; discharges—normal, pathogenic; tumors, swelling, menstruating, diaper, incontinent, infant stool-meconium, yellow, green; bloody urine, urinary dribbling, constipated stool, diarrhea, hemorrhoids, ulcerations, nodules, cysts, cracks, fissures, abscesses, lacerations, abrasions, urine and stool abnormalities—blood (red and tarry), worms, discolored, stones, undigested food; vaginal hemorrhage, bloody show, amniotic fluid, prolapse—uterine, rectal, surgical alterations

3. Clothing. Work clothes, fully clad, underclothing, naked, mod clothing, bizarre clothing, summer light clothing,

heavy winter clothing–appropriate and inappropriate to climate; heavy socks, multiple pairs of socks, gloves, business dress, uniform, nightwear–pajamas, nightgown; formal evening wear, clean, soiled, wet, buttons and zippers closed, buttons and zippers opened, diaper, bunting, cultural and national variation, religious garb, bedroom slippers, rubbers, boots, masculine clothing, feminine clothing, institutional clothing, personal clothing

4. Attachments and prostheses. Jewelry, wedding band, rings, watches, eyeglasses–bifocals, trifocals, sunglasses, tinted glasses; contact lenses, hearing aids, dentures, bridgework, bandages, dressings, slings, colostomy bag, ileostomy bag, pacemaker, artificial limbs, braces, artificial larynx, facial prostheses, catheters–chest, bladder, drains; intubation–gastric, chest, tracheostomy, gastrostomy, intestinal, rectal; dressings–heavy, absorbent, sponges, bandaid, adhesive butterfly, improvised bandage, ace bandage; support hose, support socks, heel and elbow protectors, restraints, infusions–venous, peritoneal, dialysis; monitor leads, EEG and EKG lead attachments, blood pressure cuff; crutches, canes, walkers, wheelchair, corrective shoes, urinary bag–internal, external; vaginal pads, tampons, diapers, trusses, braces–teeth, extremities, pelvic, back; sutures, casts, compresses, heating pads, hot water bottle

b. External Environment of the Client

1. Immediate: personal possession–wallet, purse, blanket, pictures, luggage, books, newspaper, letters, brief case, toilet articles, easy chair, denture cup, toys, food, drugs; room–small, large, medium; room location–health care facility, home, school, campus, industry, migrant camp, nursery, clinic, single home, townhouse, high rise apartment, home for the aged, mobile home, shack, homeless; type of room–bathroom, kitchen, living room, garage; furnishing–type, number, absence of; presence of other persons–parents, husband, wife, children, neighbors, friends, clergy, lawyer, police, other relatives, strangers, co-workers, colleagues, health care personnel, total number of persons
2. Neighborhood: urban, rural, inner city, suburbs, industrial, retirement community, college town, military installation, homeowners, rentals, young adults, river or harbor town, beach, farm, resort, paved, unpaved, lawns,

tree-lined streets, absence of shrubbery, successful stores, well-designed store fronts, deteriorated business area, many vacancies, boarded-up store fronts, flowers, shrubs, trees, lawns, dusty, litter, parks, playground; available services within one block or within walking distances—grocery store, supermarket, specialty stores, delicatesen, bakery, laundry and cleaners, bookstore, shoe repair, physician and dentist offices, schools, church, police department, fire department, ambulance service; health care facilities—outpatient and inpatient, public transportation; heavy traffic, light traffic, museums, theaters, liquor stores, cocktail lounges, bars, coffee houses, pool halls, athletic associations, bowling alleys, street lighting, emergency call system, suicide prevention center, lighted hallways, elevators, indoor plumbing, bathroom—individual, shared; refrigerator, disposal of waste—disposals, garbage cans; pets—dogs, cats, other; presence or absence of flies, rodents, mosquitos, heat, air conditioning, handrailings on stairways, rugs, wooden floors, dirt floors

II. Observations Made by Hearing

a. The Client

1. Voice and speech: calm, excited, high pitched, soprano, alto, bass, falsetto, tenor, demanding, verbal messages—expressions of need, problems, hopes, fears, concerns, attitude, pain, verbal expressions of identification and orientation, complaints and descriptions of pain—local, generalized, sharp, dull, headache, continuing, intermittent, dizziness, nausea, ringing in the ears; expressions of gratitude, disordered thought, disordered verbal content; requests for items, services, people, companionship, love, care; soft, inaudible, loud, jargon, crying, laughing, face-to-face conversation, telephone conversation, masculine, feminine, stammering, eructation, hiccough, burping, esophageal speech, unintelligible speech, talkative, strained, whispering, hoarse, stuttering, trembling, tongue-tied, slurred, lisp, gargle, groan, foreign language, snoring, aphasic, singing, grunting, silent, dialect—local, regional, national; vernacular, moaning, muffled, babbling, belching, screeching, gasping
2. Breathing: rhythmic, slow, rapid, shallow, quiet, forced, difficult inhalation, difficult exhalation, deep, stertorous, Cheyne-Stokes, apnea, wheezing, whistling, blowing, diverted through tracheostomy, coughing, sneezing, labored,

shallow, vocal vibrations, yawning, gasping, panting, rales, noisy, rattling, sighing, harsh sounds, high-pitched sounds

3. Heart sounds: apex rate–regular beat, irregular beat, tachycardia, bradycardia; murmur, absence of sound, cardiac rub, extra heart sounds; blood pressure–high, low, high diastolic
4. Abdomen: presence of peristalsis, hyperactive peristalsis, hypoactive peristalsis, absence of peristalsis, flatus

b. Environment
   1. Immediate: dripping, clicking, sucking, conversation with client and/or in the vicinity of client, traffic, public address system, laughing, absence of sounds; radio, television, phonograph sounds, noises–squeaks, banging, clanging, knocking, dishes, carts, utensils, elevators, stairs
   2. Neighborhood: traffic–heavy, light, distressful–ambulance sirens, police sirens, fire engines; trains, airplanes, car horns, animals–dogs, cats, farm animals, birds and wild animals; music–soft, rock and roll, mixed, loud, popular, live, recorded; children's voices, crying, screaming, calling, telephones, knocking, radio and television, phonograph, church bells, industrial sounds, bumping, hammering, sawing, pulling and pushing items and carts

III. Observations Made by Touching

a. The Client–body contour, size
   1. Head: hair–dry, coarse, soft, fine, baby fine; fontanels–soft, closed, bulging; lumps, swelling; forehead–warm, cold, moist
   2. Skin: smooth, clammy, rough, moist, dry, lumps, fat distribution, tumors, warts, moles, abscesses, edema, cold, cool, warm, hot; pulsations–regular, irregular, intermittent, strong, forceful, bounding, weak, scarcely perceptible, thready; goose flesh, painful, swelling
   3. Chest: expansion and relaxation, masses, painful areas, breast–lumps, engorged, size, scar, tender, absence of; pulses–brachial, carotid, radial, temporal, femoral, pedal, popliteal, facial; enlarged axillary nodes
   4. Abdomen: soft, hard, masses, tumors, distended, flat full urinary bladder, gaseous abdomen, painful, localized swelling, herniation, taut, uterine contractions, scars, palpable stool
   5. Dressings: wet, dry
   6. Bedding: wet, dry, damp, saturated, warm, cold,

smooth, rough, torn, size, absent

7. Muscle tension; muscle relaxation, throbbing, chills, twitching, spasm, convulsing, tremors, tumors, tics, firmness and fit of prostheses

b. Environment

Temperature and humidity of immediate environment, outdoor temperature and humidity; presence or absence of supports and railings, fences, bedsides

IV. Observations Made by Smelling

a. The Client

Perspiration, body odor, foot odor, axillary odor, pubic odor, hair odor—oily, perfumes, hairdressing; breath odor—sweet, alcohol, musty, tobacco, onion, garlic, commercial gargles, fetid, spicy, aromatic, pungent; bodily discharges—feces, urine, vomitus, purulent, necrotic, burned skin, burned or singed hair; use of chemicals—iodoform, liniments, ointments, anesthetics, antiseptics, deodorant, soap; absence of odors, unidentified odors

b. Environment

Food odors: vegetables, fruits, meat, charcoal pit, barbecue, condiments, spices, coffee, restaurant odor, bakery, decaying food; exhaust—traffic, industrial odors, hospital odors, burning leaves, marijuana, gas odors; odor of deodorants—pine oil, lysol, soap, peppermint; laboratory odors—antiseptics, cleaning materials, sprays; flowers, shrubs, hay, mowed lawn, farm odors, animal odors—skunk, dog, cat, horse; absence of odors, unidentified odors

• *Appendix C*
Definitions and ABCDs of Nursing Process Phases

Assessing

reviewing a situation for the purpose of diagnosing the client's problems.

Assess
By
Collecting data and
Diagnosing

Planning

determining what can be done, what goals are necessary, to assist the client.

Author the
Blueprint,
Contemplate alternatives,
Devise strategy

Implementing

performing actions necessary to achieve goals.

Actions
Basic to
Coordinating and
Delegating

Evaluating

appraising client's behavioral changes as these relate to nurse actions.

Audit
Behavior
Consistent with
Determined goals

• *Appendix D*
Application of Nursing Process—Sensory Deprivation

Assessing

Is slow in responding to questions

Does not know name initially; later remembers it

Is disoriented to time and place

Spends most of day alone

Has no radio or television

Has no calendar or clock

Is in room by self at end of hall

Bed position is such that client is unable to see out window

Has few staff contacts

Has no visitors

Does not move in bed by self unless instructed to do so

Can sit but unable to stand

Remains flat in bed at most times

Continuous humming noises heard in room from ice machine in adjacent room; bed parallel to wall where noise is most obvious

Nursing Diagnosis: Sensory Deprivation

Planning

Plan contacts by nursing staff to talk with client every hour

Use touch in getting the attention of client and to convey caring

Arrange furniture to allow client to look out window and to increase distance from wall noise

Arrange for insulation of ice machine and assure that machine does not touch wall

Transfer to 4-bed room, when available, with other clients who are alert, talkative

Play radio and choose stations that have weather and time checks, dates, various news items, music, male and female voices

Place clock and calendar within line of vision

Keep room door open

Give date, time, day of week in responding to client

Call client by name

Plan passive and active exercise every two hours

Transport to solarium or game room in A.M. and P.M. for at least ½ hour

Arrange for volunteer visitor to spend ½ hour with client in A.M. and P.M.

Implementing	Evaluating
All nursing team members are to participate in implementing strategies and collecting data concerning client's response to strategy	*Expectation:* Diminish the sensory deprivation of client; demonstration of sensory integrity by client
Client's nurse will coordinate strategies	Is more alert
Have housekeeping staff rearrange room	Initiates conversation
Have maintenance personnel move ice machine away from wall; insert insulating material at rear of machine to decrease noise	Moves and sits up in bed without direction
	Selects radio stations of interest
	Greets staff as they pass in hall and as they enter room
	Is oriented to time, place, and date
	Knows the names of three nursing staff members and the volunteer visitor
	Converses with other clients in the solarium
	Makes selection of pajamas to be worn

Yura, H: Climate to foster utilization of the nursing process. In Providing a Climate for the Utilization of Nursing Personnel. New York, National League for Nursing, 1974.

Bibliography

Books

Abdellah F, Beland I, Martin A, et al: Patient-centered Approaches to Nursing, New York, Macmillan, 1960

Aguilera D, Messick J, Farrell M: Crisis Intervention: Theory and Methodology. 2nd edition St. Louis, Mosby, 1974

Allport F: Theories of Perception and the Concept of Structure. New York, Wiley, 1955

American Nurses Association: Standards of Nursing Practice. Kansas City, American Nurses Association, 1973

Anderson B: The Psychology Experiment, second edition. Belmont, Calif, Brooks/Cole, 1971

Ardrey R: The Territorial Imperative. New York, Atheneum, 1966

Bailey JT, Claus KE: Decision Making in Nursing. St. Louis, Mosby, 1975

Banathy BH: Instructional Systems. Fearon, Palo Alto, California, 1968

Barnard C: The Functions of the Executive. Cambridge, Harvard University Press, 1964

Becknell EP, Smith DM: System of Nursing Practice–A Clinical Nursing Assessment Tool. Philadelphia, Davis, 1975

Benedikter H: The Nursing Audit–A Necessity. How Shall it be Done? (Publication No. 20–1501) New York, National League for Nursing, 1973

Bermosk LS, Mordan MJ: Interviewing in Nursing. New York, Macmillan, 1964

Bertalanffy L von: General System Theory. New York, George Braziller, 1968

Bevis EO: Curriculum Building in Nursing–A Process. St. Louis, Mosby, 1973

Bloom BS, Hastings JT, Madaus GF: Handbook on Formative and Summative Evaluation of Student Learning. New York, McGraw-Hill, 1971

Bonney V, Rothberg J: Nursing Diagnosis and Therapy–An Instrument for Evaluation and Measurement. New York, The League Exchange, National League for Nursing, 1963

Braden CJ, Herban NL: Community Health–A Systems Approach. New York, Appleton-Century-Crofts, 1976

Branch MF, Paxton PP (eds): Providing Safe Nursing Care for Ethnic People of Color. New York, Appleton-Century-Crofts, 1976

Brook RH: Quality of Care Assessment: Comparison of Two Methods of Peer Review. Bethesda Md., U.S. Department of Health, Education and Welfare, No. HRA–74–3100, July 1973

Brown BB: New Mind, New Body. New York, Bantam, 1974

Brown EL: Nursing For the Future. New York, Russell Sage Foundation, 1948

———: Newer Dimensions of Patient Care, parts 1, 2, and 3. New York, Russell Sage Foundation, 1964

Brown M, Fowler G: Psychodynamic Nursing, 4th edition. Philadelphia, Saunders, 1971

Buber M: The Knowledge of Man. New York, Harper & Row, 1965

———: I and Thou, 2nd edition. New York, Scribner's, 1958

Buckley W (ed): Modern Systems Research for the Behavioral Scientist. Chicago, Aldine, 1968

Byers V: Nursing Observation. Dubuque, Ia., Brown, 1968

Catholic Hospital Association. Ethical Issues in Nursing–A Proceedings. St. Louis, Catholic Hospital Association, 1976

Catholic Hospital Association. Religious Aspects of Medical Care: A Handbook of Religious Practices of All Faiths. St. Louis, Catholic Hospital Association, 1975

Conley VC: Curriculum and Instruction in Nursing. Boston, Little, Brown, 1973

Copi I: Introduction to Logic, 2nd Edition. New York, Macmillan, 1961

Davidson SVS (ed). PDTO Utilization and Audit in Patient Care. St. Louis, Mosby, 1976

Davis F (ed): The Nursing Profession: Five Sociological Essays. New York, Wiley, 1966

Douglass L, Bevis EO: Nursing leadership in action. St. Louis, Mosby, 1974

Dubos R: Man Adapting. New Haven, Yale University Press, 1965

Dunn HL: High-Level Wellness. Arlington, Va., Beatty, 1967

Einstein A, Infeld L: The Evolution of Physics. New York, Simon and Schuster, 1938

Erikson EH: Childhood and Society, 2nd edition, New York, Norton, 1963

Fast J: Body Language. New York, Evans, 1970

Fivars G, Gosnell D: Nursing Evaluation: The Problem and the Process. New York, Macmillan, 1966

Flexner A: Universities. New York, Oxford University Press, 1930

Folta J, Deck E (eds): A Sociological Framework for Patient Care. New York, Wiley, 1966

Fowkes, WC, Hunn VK: Clinical Assessment For the Nurse Practitioner. St. Louis, Mosby, 1973

Fox DJ: Fundamentals of Research in Nursing. 3rd Edition, New York, Appleton-Century-Crofts, 1976

Frances G, Munjas B: Manual of Social Psychologic Assessment. New York, Appleton-Century-Crofts, 1976.

Frank CM: Foundations of Nursing. Philadelphia, Saunders, 1959, p 78

Frankenburg WK, Dodds JB: Denver Developmental Screening Test Manual. Denver, Ladoca Project and Publishing Foundation, 1970

Frankl V: Man's Search for Meaning. New York, Washington Square Press, 1963

Freeman RB (ed.), Family Coping Index. Developed by Johns Hopkins School of Hygiene and Public Health and Richmond Instructive Visiting Nurse Association—City Health Department, Nursing Service (Richmond-Hopkins Cooperative Nursing Study), 1964

Froebe DJ, Bain RJ: Quality Assurance Programs and Controls in Nursing. St. Louis, Mosby, 1976

Fromm E: The Art of Loving. New York, Harper & Row, 1956

Gebbie KM, Lavin MA: Classification of Nursing Diagnoses, St. Louis, Mosby, 1975

Gebbie KM (ed): Summary of the Second National Conference—Classification of Nursing Diagnosis. St. Louis, Clearinghouse—National Group for Classification of Nursing Diagnoses, 1976

Gillies DA, Alyn IB: Patient Assessment and Management by the Nurse Practitioner. Philadelphia, Saunders, 1976

Goble FG: The Third Force. New York, Grossman, 1970

Grace-Reynolds Health Care Trust Grant to Grace Hospital, Inc. E. Louise Clark, principal investigator, 1976

Griffiths D: Administrative Theory. New York, Appleton-Century-Crofts, 1959

Halpert HP, Horvath, W, Young JP: An Administrator's Handbook on the Application of Operations Research to the Management of Mental Health Systems. National Clearinghouse for Mental Health Information. No. 1003, 1970

Halpin A (e): Administrative Theory in Education. New York. Macmillan, 1958

Hardy ME (ed): Theoretical Foundations for Nursing. New York, MSS Information Corporation, 1973

Harmer B: Methods and Principles of Teaching the Principles and Practice of Nursing. New York, Macmillan, 1926

Harms M: Components of a conceptual framework. In Pathways to Practice, vol. 2. To Serve the Future Hour. B. B. Heitt (ed). Atlanta, Southern Regional Education Board, 1974

Haussmann RKD, Hegyvary ST, Newman JF: Monitoring Quality of Nursing Care, Part II: Assessment and Study of Correlates. Bethesda, Md. U. S. Department of Health, Education, and Welfare, July, 1976

Henderson V: The Nature of Nursing. New York, Macmillan, 1966

Hurst J, Walker HK (eds): The Problem-Oriented System. New York, Medcom, 1972

Jaco E: Patients, Physicians and Illness. Glencoe, Ill., Free Press, 1958

Jacox AK, Norris CM: Organizing For Independent Nursing Practice. New York, Appleton-Century-Crofts, 1977

Jaeger D, Simmons L: The Aged Ill. New York, Appleton-Century-Crofts, 1970

Jelinek RC, Haussmann RKD, Hegyvary ST, Newman J: A Methodology for Monitoring Quality of Nursing Care. Bethesda, Md. U.S. Department of Health, Education, and Welfare, 1974

Johnson M, Davis MI, Bilitch M: Problem-Solving in Nursing Practice. Dubuque, Ia., Brown, 1970

Jourard SM: The Transparent Self. Princeton, N.J., Van Nostrand, 1964

King IM: Toward a Theory for Nursing. New York, Wiley, 1971

Kinlein ML: Independent Nursing Practice With Clients. Philadelphia, Lippincott, 1977

Kintzel K (ed): Advanced Concepts in Clinical Nursing, 2nd edition. Philadelphia, Lippincott, 1977

Kramer M: Reality Shock—Why Nurses Leave Nursing. St. Louis, Mosby, 1974

Kron T: Communication in Nursing. Philadelphia, Saunders, 1972

Kuethe J: The Teaching–Learning Process. Glenview, Ill., Scott, Freeman, 1968

Lachman S: The Foundation of Science, New York, Vantage, 1960

Larkin PD, Backer BA: Problem-Oriented Nursing Assessment. New York, McGraw-Hill, 1977

Leavell H, Clark EG: Preventive Medicine for the Doctor in His Community, 31st edition. New York, McGraw-Hill, 1966

Lee W: Decision Theory and Human Behavior. New York, Wiley, 1971

Levine MF: Introduction to Clinical Nursing. Philadelphia, Davis, 1973

Lewis G: Nurse-Patient Communication, second edition. Dubuque, Ia., Brown, 1973

Lewis L, Carozza V, Carroll M, et al: Defining Clinical Content Graduate Nursing Programs, Medical-Surgical Nursing. Boulder, Colorado. Western Interstate Commission for Higher Education, February, 1967

Lewis L: Planning Patient Care. Dubuque, Ia., Brown, 1970

Little DE, Carnevali DL: Nursing Care Planning, 2nd edition. Philadelphia, Lippincott, 1969

Luce GG: Body Time. New York, Bantam, 1971

Lysaught J: Abstract for Action. New York, McGraw-Hill, 1970

Mager R: Goal Analysis. Belmont, Calif., Fearson, 1972

———: Preparing Instructional Objectives. Belmont, Calif., Fearon, 1962

Maloney E, Verdisco L, Shortridge L: How to Collect and Record a Health History. Philadelphia, Lippincott, 1976

Maslow AH: Toward A Psychology of Being, 2nd edition. Princeton, N. J., Van Nostrand, 1968

———: Motivation and Personality, 2nd edition. New York, Harper & Row, 1970

Mayeroff M: On Caring. New York, Harper & Row, 1971

Mayers MA: A Systematic Approach to the Nursing Care Plan. New York, Appleton-Century-Crofts, 1972

McAllister JB: A Syllabus of Logic. Washington, DC, The Catholic University of America, 1942

McCaffery M: Nursing Management of the Patient with Pain. Philadelphia, Lippincott, 1972

McCarthy, DG (ed): Responsible Stewardship of Human Life-Inquiries into Medical Ethics II. St. Louis, The Catholic Hospital Association, 1976

McKay, RP: The Process of Theory Development in Nursing. New York. Teachers College, Columbia University, A Report of an Ed D Doctoral Project, 1965

Metheny N, Snively WD: Nurses' Handbook of Fluid Balance. Philadelphia, Lippincott, 1967

Meyer B, Heidgerken LE: Introduction to Research in Nursing. Philadelphia, Lippincott, 1962

Montagu A: On Being Human, New York, Hawthorn, 1966

———: The Direction of Human Development. New York, Hawthorn, 1970

———: Touching—The Human Significance of the Skin. New York, Harper & Row, 1971

Moody R: Life After Life. New York, Bantam, 1975

Murphy JF (ed): Theoretical Issues in Professional Nursing, New York, Appleton-Century-Crofts, 1971

Murray R, Zentner J: Nursing Assessment and Health Promotion Through the Life Span. Englewood Cliffs, N. J., Prentice-Hall, 1975

———: Nursing Concepts for Health Promotion. Englewood Cliffs, N. J., Prentice-Hall, 1975

National Commission for the Study of Nursing and Nursing Education, Inc: Action in Nursing: Progress in Professional Purpose, New York, McGraw-Hill, 1974

National League for Nursing: Evaluation—The Whys and The Ways. New York, The National League for Nursing, 1965

National League for Nursing: Problem-oriented Systems of Patient Care. New York, National League for Nursing, 1974

National League for Nursing: Quality Assurance—A Joint Venture, New York, National League for Nursing, 1975

National League for Nursing: Quality Assurance: Models for Nursing Education. New York, National League for Nursing, 1976

National League for Nursing: Quest for Quality: A Self Evaluation Guide to Patient Care. Prepared by Committee on Quality of Patient Care. Department of Hospital Nursing. New York, National League for Nursing, 1966

Newell A, Simon H: Human Problem Solving. Englewood Cliffs, N. J., Prentice-Hall, 1972

Nightingale F: Notes on Nursing: What It Is and What It Is Not. A facsimile of the first edition published in 1859. Philadelphia, Lippincott, 1946

Nordmark M, Rohweder A: Science Foundations of Nursing. Philadelphia, Lippincott, 1967

Nursing Development Conference Group: Concept Formalization in Nursing—Process and Product. Boston, Little, Brown, 1973

Orem DE: Nursing: Concepts of Practice. New York, McGraw-Hill, 1971

Orlando IJ: The Dynamic Nurse–Patient Relationship. New York, Putnam's, 1961

O'Rourke KD (ed): The Mission of Healing-Readings in Christian Values and Health Care. St. Louis, The Catholic Hospital Association, 1974

Ozimek D, Yura H: Who is the Nurse Practitioner? New York, National League for Nursing, 1975

Paterson JG, Zderad LT: Humanistic Nursing. New York, Wiley, 1976

Peplau HE: Theory: The professional dimension. In Proceedings of the First Nursing Theory Conference, March 20–21, 1969, edited by Catherine M. Norris, Kansas City, Ka., University of Kansas Medical Center, 1969

Phaneuf MC: The Nursing Audit—Profile for Excellence. New York, Appleton-Century-Crofts, 1972

———: The Nursing Audit—Self Regulation in Nursing Practice, 2nd edition. New York, Appleton-Century-Crofts, 1976

Pohl M: Teaching Function of the Nursing Practitioner. Dubuque, Ia., Brown, 1968

Public Law 92–603, 92nd Congress, HRI, October 30, 1972

Quest for Quality: A Self Evaluation Guide to Patient Care. New York, National League for Nursing, 1966 (No. 20–1212)

Quality Assurance: Models for Nursing Education. New York, National League for Nursing, 1976 (No. 15–1611)

Quality Assurance of Medical Care-Monograph-Regional Medical Programs Service, Health Services and Mental Health Administration, Bethesda, Md., US Department of Health, Education, and Welfare, No. (HSM) 73–7021, February, 1973

Raiffa H: Decision Analysis. Reading, Mass., Addison-Wesley, 1970

Riehl, JP, Roy C: Conceptual Models for Nursing Practice. New York, Appleton-Century-Crofts, 1974

Rogers ME: Nursing Science: Introduction to the Theoretical Basis of Nursing. Philadelphia, Davis, 1970

Roy C: Introduction to Nursing: An Adaptation Model. Englewood Cliffs, N. J., Prentice-Hall, 1976

Samuels M, Bennett H: The Well Body Book. New York, Random House, 1973

Schein E (ed): Professional Education: Some New Directions. Carnegie Commission on Higher Education. New York, McGraw-Hill, 1972

Selye H: Stress Without Distress. Philadelphia, Lippincott, 1974

Sigma Theta Tau: First Regional Conference. The Assessment of Leader Behaviors, Storrs, Connecticut, Sigma Theta Tau, 1969

Simon H: The Sciences of the Artificial. Cambridge, The MIT Press, 1969

Skipper JK, Leonard RC (ed): Social Interaction and Patient Care. Philadelphia, Lippincott, 1965

Smith DW: Medical-Surgical Nursing in the Curriculum—Purpose and Process, Curriculum and Instruction in Medical Surgical and Psychiatric Nursing in Baccalaureate Programs. Edited by V. Conley, Washington, DC, The Catholic University of America Press, 1970

Straub KM, Parker KS (ed): Continuity of Patient Care: The Role of Nursing. Proceedings of the Workshop. Washington, DC, The Catholic University of America Press, 1966

Sutterly D, Donnelly G: Meeting nursing needs throughout the life cycle, chapter 3. In: Kintzel K (ed): Advanced Concepts in Clinical Nursing. Philadelphia, Lippincott, 1971

Schwartz R (ed): Perceiving, Sensing, and Knowing. Garden City, N.Y., Anchor, 1965

Taylor DB: A clinical information system: a tool for improving nurses' decisions in planning patient care. In: ANA Clinical Sessions. New York, Appleton-Century-Crofts, 1970

Toffler A: Future Shock. New York, Random House, 1970

Torres G: Educational Trends and the integrated approach to curriculum. In: Faculty-Curriculum Development, Part 4: Unifying the Curriculum—The Integrated Approach. (Publication No. 15–1522) New York, National League for Nursing, 1974

Torres G, Yura H: Today's Conceptual Framework: Its Relationship to the Curriculum Development Process. New York, National League for Nursing, 1974

Toward Quality in Nursing, Needs and Goals. Washington DC, Public Health Service, US Department of Health, Education and Welfare, 1963

Travelbee J: Interpersonal Aspects of Nursing, 2nd edition. Philadelphia, Davis, 1971

Tucker SM, et al: Patient Care Standards. St. Louis, Mosby, 1975

Ujhely GB: Determinants of the Nurse–Patient Relationship. New York, Springer, 1968

Vernon M: Perception Through Experience. London, Methuen, 1970

Walker V: Nursing and Ritualistic Practice. New York, Macmillan 1967

Wandelt MA: Guide for the Beginning Researcher. New York, Appleton-Century-Crofts, 1970

Wandelt MA, Agar JW: Quality Patient Care Scale. New York, Appleton-Century-Crofts, 1974

Wandelt MA, Stewart DS: Slater Nursing Competencies Rating Scale. New York, Appleton-Century-Crofts, 1975

Webster's Third International Dictionary. Springfield, Mass., Merriam, 1967

Weed L: Medical Records, Medical Education, and Patient Care. Cleveland Press of Case Western Reserve University, 1970

Wensley E: Nursing Service Without Walls—A Call to Action to

All Communities Coast to Coast. New York, National League for Nursing, 1963

Wiedenbach E: Clinical Nursing: A Helping Art. New York, Springer, 1964

Worrell J: Nursing implication in the care of the patient experiencing sensory deprivation. In: Kintzel K (ed): Advanced Concepts in Clinical Nursing. Philadelphia, Lippincott, 1971

Yura H: Climate to foster utilization of the nursing process. In: Providing a Climate for the Utilization of Nursing Personnel. New York, National League for Nursing, 1975

Yura H, Ozimek D, Walsh MB: Nursing Leadership: Theory and Process. New York, Appleton-Century-Crofts, 1976

Zborowski M: People in Pain. San Francisco, Jossey-Boss, 1969

Zderad L, Belcher H: Developing Behavioral Concepts in Nursing. Atlanta, Southern Regional Education Board, 1968

Periodicals

Abdellah FG, Levine E: Polling patients and personnel, Part I. What patients say about their nursing care. Hospitals 31:44–48, November 1, 1957

Abdellah FG: Criterion measures in nursing. Nurs Res 10:21–26, winter 1961

Abdellah FG: The nature of nursing science. Nurs Res 18:390–393, September–October 1969

Agree BC: Beginning an independent nursing practice. Am J Nurs 74:636–642, April 1974

Alexander M, Brown M: Physical exam, Part 2: history taking. Nurs '73 3:35–39, August 1973

Alfano G: The Loeb Center for Nursing and Rehabilitation—a professional approach to nursing practice. Nurs Clin N Am 4:487–493, September 1969

Allekian C: Intrusion of territory and personal space: an anxiety-inducing factor for hospitalized persons—an exploratory study. Nurs Res 22:236–241, May–June 1973

Amacher NJ: Tough is a way of caring. Am J Nurs 73:852–854, May 1973

American Journal of Nursing: Establishing standards for nursing practice (unsigned). 69:1458–63

American Nurses' Association: Code for Nurses. The American Nurse. Kansas City, Mo., October 15, 1976

American Nurses' Association's First Position on Education for Nursing. Am J Nurs 65:106–111, December 1965

ANA peer review criteria mandated by HEW Contract (News). Nurs Outlook 22:545, September 1974

ANA Convention '76. Am J Nurs 75:1123–1138, July 1976

Anderson MD, Pleticha JM: Emergency unit patients' perceptions of stressful life events. Nurs Res 23:378–383, September–October 1974

Angus M: Evaluation: a constructive or a destructive force? Can Nurs 62:26–28, July 1966

Anonymous. Notes of a Dying Professor. Nurs Outlook 20:502–506, August 1972

Aradine CR, Guthneck M: The problem-oriented record in a family health service. Am J Nurs 74:1108–1112, June 1974

Arnold HM: I—Thou. Am J Nurs 70:2554–2556, December 1970

Aspinall MJ: Development of a patient-completed admission questionnaire and its comparison with the nursing interview. Nurs Res 24:377–381, September–October 1975

Aspinall MJ: Nursing diagnosis—the weak link. Nurs Outlook 24:433–436, July 1976

Backscheider JE: Self-care requirements, self-care capabilities, and nursing systems in the diabetic nurse management clinic. Am J Public Health 64:1138–1146, December, 1974

Bailey DE: Clinical inference in nursing: Analysis of nursing action patterns. Nurs Res 16:154–160, spring 1967

Bailey JT, McDonald FJ, Claus KE: Evaluation of the development of creative behavior in an experimental nursing program. Nurs Res 19:100–108, March–April 1970

Bailit H, Lewis J, Hockheiser L, Bush N: Assessing the quality of care. Nurs Outlook 23:153–159, March 1975

Barckley V: Enough time for good nursing. Nurs Outlook 12:44–48, April 1964

Barrett–Lennard GT: Significant aspects of a helping relationship. Canad Ment Health (Spec Suppl) 47:1–5, 1965

Bates B, Kern MS: Doctor–nurse teamwork: what helps? what hinders? Am J Nurs 67:2066–2071, October 1967

Bates B, Lynaugh J: Teaching physical assessment. Nurs Outlook 23:297–302, May 1975

Bayer M: Community diagnosis—through sense, sight, and sound. Nurs Outlook 21:712–713, November 1973

Berg H: Nursing audit and outcome criteria. Nurs Clin N A 9:331–335, June 1974

Binzley V: State: overlooked factor in newborn nursing. Am J Nurs 77:102–103, January 1977

Bishop B: A guide to assessing parenting capabilities. Am J Nurs 76:1784–1787, November 1976

Black, Sister Kathleen: Social isolation and the nursing process. Nurs Clin North Am 8:575–586, December 1973

Blau K: It's the patient's problem—and decision. Nurs Outlook 19:587–589, September 1971

Bloch D: Some crucial terms in nursing: what do they really mean? Nurs Outlook 22:689–694, November 1974

———: Evaluation of nursing care in terms of process and outcome: Issues in research and quality assurance. Nurs Res 24:256–263, July–August 1975

Bloom JT, et al: Problem-oriented charting. Am J Nurs 71:2144–2148, November 1971

Bonkowsky ML: Problem-oriented medical records: Adapting the POMR to community child health care. Nurs Outlook 20:515–518, August 1972

Brimigion J, Miller DB: Nursing administration in long-term care facilities: a dual-kardex system. J Nurs Administr 1:26–30, March–April 1971

Brodt DE: Obstacles to individualized patient care. Nurs Outlook 14:35–36, December 1966

———: A synergistic theory of nursing. Am J Nurs 69:1674–1676, August 1969

Brown MI: Research in the development of nursing theory. Nurs Res 13:109–112, spring 1964

Brown MI: Social theory in geriatric nursing research. Nurs Res 17:213–217, May–June 1968

Brown MM: The epidemiologic approach to the study of clinical nursing diagnosis. Nurs Forum 13(4):346–359, 1974

Bullough B: The medicare-medicaid amendments. Am J Nurs 73:1926–1929, November 1973

Burgess A, Burns J: Why patients seek care. Am J Nurs 73:314–316, February 1973

Burnside IM: Touching is talking. Am J Nurs 73:2060–2063, December 1973

Burrill M: Helping students identify and solve patients' problems. Nurs Outlook 14:46–48, February 1966

Butler HJ, Flood FR: Evaluating nursing care in mental hospital. Am J Nurs 62:84–85, August 1962

Calnan MF, Hanron JB: Patient-centered communication. Superv Nurse 2:67–71, February 1971

Campbell MA: Identifying nursing problems. Can Nurse 61:96–99, February 1965

Carlson S: A practice approach to the nursing process. Am J Nurs 72:1589–1591, September 1972

Carn I: The nursing audit as a learning tool for undergraduates in a community nursing service. Nurs Clin N Am 4:351–358, June 1969

Carnegie ME: The research attitude begins on the undergraduate level. Nurs Res 23:99, March–April 1974

Carrieri VK, Sitzman J: Components of the nursing process. Nurs Clin N Am 6:115–124, March 1971

Chambers W: Nursing diagnosis. Am J Nurs 62:102–104, November, 1962

Changing Times: The stormy 70's—big changes still to come, (unsigned) 26:25–31, 1972

Chater SS: A conceptual framework for curriculum development. Nurs Outlook 23:428–433, July 1975

Chopoorian T, Craig MM: PL 93–641 Nursing and health care delivery. Am J Nurs 76:1988–1991, December 1976

Chrisman M: Dyspnea. Am J Nurs 74:643–646, April 1974

Cinca R: Over the years with the nursing care plan. Nurs Outlook 20:706–711, November 1972

Clark EL, Diggs WW: Quantifying patient care needs. Hospitals 45(18):96, 1971

Cleary F: A theoretical model: its potential for adaptation to nursing. Image 41(1):14–20, 1971

Cleland V: Nursing research and graduate education. Nurs Outlook 23:642–645, October 1975

Clissold GK, Metz EA: Evaluation—a tangible process. Nurs Outlook 14:41–45, March 1966

Cochran C, Hansen PJ: Developing an evaluation tool by group action. Am J Nurs 62:94–97, March 1962

Coladarci AP: What about that word profession? Am J Nurs 63:116–118, October 1963

Condon MB: Teaching the teachers. Nurs Outlook 19:804–806, December 1971

Cornell SA, Brush F: Systems approach to nursing care plans. Am J Nurs 71:1376–1378, July 1971

Craven RF: Primary health care practice in the nursing home. Am J Nurs 76:1958–1960, December 1976

Crosby MH: Control systems and children with lymphoblastic leukemia. Nurs Clin N Am 6:407–413, September 1971

Cullen PB: Patients with colorectal cancer: how to assess and meet their needs. Nurs '76 6:42–47, September 1976

Dahlin B: Rehabilitation and the assessment of patient need. Nurs Clin N Am 1:375–386, September 1966

Daubenmire MJ, King D: Nursing process models: a systems approach. Nurs Outlook 21:512–517, August 1973

Daubert EA: A system to evaluate home health care services. Nurs Outlook 25:168–171, March 1977

Davitz LJ, Pendleton SH: Nurses' inferences of suffering. Nurs Res 18:100–107, March–April 1969

Davitz L, Sameshima Y, Davitz J: Suffering as viewed in six different cultures. Am J Nurs 76:1296–1297, August, 1976

De Geyndt W: Five approaches for assessing the quality of care. Hosp Admin 15:21–42, winter 1970

De Tornay R: Measuring problem-solving skills by means of the simulated clinical nursing problem test. J Nurs Educ 7(3):3, 1968

Dickoff J, James P: A theory of theories: A position paper. Nurs Res 17:197–203, May–June 1968

———: Researching research's role in theory development. Nurs Res 17:204–206, May–June 1968

Dickoff J, James P, Wiedenbach E: Theory in a practice discipline, Part I. Practice oriented theory. Nurs Res 17:415–435, September–October 1968

———: Theory in a practice discipline, Part II. Practice oriented research. Nurs Res 17:545–554, November–December 1968

Dickoff J, James P: Beliefs and values: bases for curriculum design. Nurs Res 19:415–427, September–October 1970

Dickoff J, James P, Semradek J: 8-4 Research, Part I: a stance for nursing research-tenacity or inquiry. Nurs Res 24:84–88, March–April 1975

———: Part II: Designing nursing research—eight points of encounter. Nurs Res 24:164–176, May–June 1975

Diers D: Applications of research to nursing practice. Image 5(2):7–11, 1972

Dietrich BJ, Miller DI: Nursing leadership—a theoretical approach. Nurs Outlook 14:52–55, August 1966

Dingle JH: The ills of man. Sci Am 229:76–84, September 1973

Donabedian A: Patient care evaluation. Hospitals 44(7):131, 1970

Donohue MA: The I—thou relationship. Nurs Outlook 14:59–61, August 1966

Donovan H: The personalized nursing audit. Superv Nurse 2: 37–41, December 1971

Doona ME: The judgment process in nursing. Image 8(2):27–29, June 1976

Downs FS, Fitzpatrick JJ: Preliminary investigations of the reliability and validity of a tool for the assessment of body position and motor activity. Nurs Res 25:404–408, November–December 1976

Doxiadis CA: Man and the space around him. Saturday Review 21–23, December 14, 1968

Drucker PF: The effective decision. Harvard Business Review 45:92–98, January–February 1967

Dubos R: Man overadapting to the environment. Psychol Today 4:50–54, 1971

Duffey M, Muhlenkamp AF: A framework for theory analysis. Nurs Outlook 22:570–574, September 1974

Dunn MA: Development of an instrument to measure nursing performance. Nurs Res 19:502–510, November–December 1970

Durand M, Prince R: Nursing Diagnosis: process and decision. Nurs Forum 5(4):50–64, 1966

Eddy L, Westbrook L, Hirsch IL: Multidisciplinary retrospective patient care audit. AM J Nurs 75:961–963, June 1975

Ellis GL: Communications and interdepartmental relationships. Nurs Forum 5(4):82–89, 1966

Ellis R: Characteristics of significant theories. Nurs Res 17: 217–222, May–June 1968

———: The practitioner as theorist. Am J Nurs 69:1434–1438, July 1969

Eriksson K: Nursing-skilled work or a profession? Inter Nurs Review 23:118–120, July–August 1976

Felton G: Increasing the quality of nursing care by introducing the concept of primary nursing: a model project. Nurs Res 24:27–32, January–February 1975

Flanagan J: The critical incident technique. Psychol Bull 51:327–358, 1954

Folta JR: Conference on the nature of science and nursing: perspectives of an applied scientist. Nurs Res 17:502–505, November–December 1968

Francis GM: Cancer: the emotional component. Am J Nurs 69: 1677–1681, August 1969

Fredette S: The art of applying theory to practice. Am J Nurs 74:856–859, May 1974

Fuller D, Rosenaur JA: A patient assessment guide. Nurs Outlook 22:460–462, July 1974

Garant C: A basis for care. Am J Nurs 72:699–701, April 1972

Gebbie KM, Lavin MA: Classifying nursing diagnoses. Am J Nurs 74:250–253, February 1974

Geitgey DA: A guide to nursing care. Nurs Outlook 17:48–49, August 1969

Giblin EC (ed): Symposium on assessment as part of the nursing process. Nurs Clin N Am 6:113–114, March 1971

Gilbo D: Nursing assessment of circulatory function. Nurs Clin N Am 3:53–64, March 1968

Gold H, Jackson M, Sachs B, Van Miter MJ: Peer review—a working experiment. Nurs Outlook 21:634–636, October 1973

Goodwin JO, Edwards BS: Developing a computer program to assist the nursing process: Phase I—from systems analysis to an expandable program. Nurs Res 24:299–305, July–August 1975

Gordon M: Assessing activity tolerance. Am J Nurs 76:72–75, January 1976

———: Nursing diagnoses and the diagnostic process. Am J Nurs 76:1298–1300, August 1976

Gortner SR: Scientific accountability in nursing. Nurs Outlook 22:764–768, December 1974

———: Research for a practice profession. Nurs Res 24: 193–197, May–June 1975

Gosnell DJ: An assessment tool to identify pressure sores. Nurs Res 22:55–59, January–February 1973

Gowan MO: Administration of college and university programs in nursing, from the viewpoint of nurse education. Proceedings of the Workshop on Administration of College Programs in Nursing. Washington, DC, The Catholic University of America Press, 1944

Grant MM, Kubo WM: Assessing a patient's hydration status. Am J Nurs 75:1306–1311, August 1975

Greenough K: Determining standards for nursing care. Am J Nurs 68:2153–2157, October 1968

Grier M: Decision making about patient care. Nurs Res 25:105–110, March–April 1976

Grier M: Hair care for the black patient. Am J Nurs 76:1781, November 1976

Griffith EW: Nursing process: a patient with a respiratory dysfunction. Nurs Clin N Am 6:145–154, March 1971

Gruis ML, Innes B: Assessment: essential to prevent pressure sores. Am J Nurs 76:1762–1764, November 1976

Gulbrandsen MW: Guide to health assessment. Am J Nurs 76:1276–1277, August 1976

Hadley BJ: Evolution of a conception of nursing. Nurs Res 18: 400–405, September–October 1969

———: Current concepts of wellness and illness: their relevance for nursing. Image 6:21–27, February 1974

Haferkorn V: Assessing individual learning needs as a basis for patient teaching. Nurs Clin N Am 6:199–209, March 1971

Hagen E: Appraising the quality of nursing care. In: American Nurses Association Eighth Nursing Research Conference held at Albuquerque, New Mexico, March 15–17, 1972. New York, American Nurses' Association, 1972, pp 1–7

Hagopian G, Kilpack V: Baccalaureate students learn assessment skills. Nurs Outlook 22:454–456, July 1974

Hall LE: Quality of Nursing Care. Address at meeting of Department of Baccalaureate and Higher Degree Programs of the New Jersey League for Nursing, February 7, 1955, Seton Hall University, Newark, New Jersey. Published in Public Health News, New Jersey State Department of Health, June 1955

———: A center for nursing. Nurs Outlook 11:805–806, November 1963

———: The Loeb Center for Nursing and Rehabilitation, Montefiore Hospital and Medical Center, Bronx, New York. Int J Nurs Studies 6(2):81–97, 1969

———: Another view of nursing care and quality. Maryland Nursing News (Spring), 1968, pp 2–12

Hamdi ME, Hutelmyer CM: A study of the effectiveness of an assessment tool in the identification of nursing care problems. Nurs Res 19:354–359, July–August 1970

Hamilton C, Pratt MK, Groen M: The nurse's active role in assessment. Nurs Clin N Am 4:249–262, June 1969

Hammond KR: Clinical inference in nursing—a psychologist's viewpoint. Nurs Res 15:27–38, winter 1966

Hammond KR, Kelly KJ, Schneider RJ, Vancini M: Clinical inference in nursing-analyzing cognitive tasks representative of nursing problems. Nurs Res 15:134–138, spring 1966

———: Clinical inference in nursing—information units used. Nurs Res 15:236–243, summer 1966

Hammond KR, Kelly KJ, Castellan NJ Jr, Schneider RJ, Vancini M: Clinical inference in nursing: use of information-seeking strategies. Nurs Res 15:330–336, fall 1966

Hammond KR, Kelly KJ, Schneider RJ, Vancini M; Clinical inference in nursing: revising judgments. Nurs Res 16:38–45, winter 1967

Hanlon JH: Theory and the practice of nursing. J Contin Educ in Nurs 5:12–18, November–December 1974

Hanna K: Nursing audit at a community hospital. Nurs Outlook 24:33–37, January 1976

Hardy ME: Theories: components, development, evaluation. Nurs Res 23:100–107, March–April 1974

Harris MI: Theory building in nursing—a review of the literature. Image 4(1):6–10, 1971

Harrison C: Deliberative nursing process versus automatic nurse action. Nurs Clin N Am 1:387–397, September 1966

Hauser MA: Initiation into peer review. Am J Nurs 75:2204–2207, December 1975

Haussmann RKD, Hegyvary ST: Field testing the nursing quality monitoring methodology: Phase II. Nurs Res 25:324–331, September–October 1976

Hazzard ME: An overview of systems theory. Nurs Clin N Am 6:385–393, September 1971

Healy EE, McGurk W: Effectiveness and acceptance of nurses' notes. Nurs Outlook 14:32–34, March 1966

Hefferin EA, Hunter RE: Nursing Assessment and care plan statements. Nurs Res 24:360–366, September–October 1975

Heinemann E, Estes N: Assessing alcoholic patients. Am J Nurs 76:785–789, May 1976

Henderson V: The nature of nursing. Am J Nurs 64:62–68, August 1964

———: Excellence in nursing. Am J Nurs 69:2133–2137, October 1969

———: On nursing care plans and their history. Nurs Outlook 21:378–379, June 1973

Hewitt HE, Pesznecker BL: Blocks to communicating with patients. Am J Nurs 64:101–103, July 1964

Hicks AP, Ashby DJ: Teaching discharge planning. Nurs Outlook 24:306–308, May 1976

Hilger EE: Developing nursing outcome criteria. Nurs Clin N Am 9:323–330, June 1974

Hirschfeld MJ: The cognitively impaired older adult. Am J Nurs 76:1981–1984, December 1976

Hitchcock JM: Crisis intervention. Am J Nurs 73:1388–1390, August 1973

Hodges LC: Systems and nursing care of the cardiac surgical patient. Nurs Clin N Am 6:415–424, September 1971

Hodgman EC: Conceptual framework to guide nursing curriculum. Nurs Forum 12:(2):110, 1973

Hoffman GS: The concept of love. Nurs Clin N Am 4:663–671, December 1969

Hogan AI: The role of the nurse in meeting the needs of the new mother. Nurs Clin N Am 3:337–344, June 1968

Holmstrom LL, Burgess AW: Assessing trauma in the rape victim AM J Nurs 75:1288–1291, August 1975

Horn RE: Information mapping: new tool to overcome the paper mountain. Educ Tech 14(5):5, 1974

Hornung GJ: Nursing diagnosis—an exercise in judgment. Nurs Outlook 4:29–30, January 1956

House MJ: Devising a care plan you can really use. Nurs '75 5:12–14, July 1975

Houser D: What to do first when a patient complains of chest pain. Nurs '76 6:54–56, November 1976

Huang SH: Nursing assessment in planning care for a diabetic patient. Nurs Clin N Am 6:135–143, March 1971

Hykawy E: A problem solving approach. Can Nurse 63:35–38, August 1967

ICN Code of Ethics for nursing. Am J Nurs 73:1351, August 1973

Jackson EB: In the screening clinic, guidelines to the appraisal of some common problems. AM J Nurs 72:1398–1400, August 1972

Jacobansky A: Strokes. Am J. Nurs 72:1260–1263, July 1972

Jacobson M: Qualitative data as a potential source of theory in nursing. Image 4(1):10–14, 1971

Jacox A: Theory construction in nursing: an overview. Nurs Res 23:4–13, January–February 1974

Joel L, Davis S: A proposal for base line data collection for psychiatric care. Persp in Psych Care 11(2):48–58, 1973

Johnson DE: The nature of a science of nursing. Nurs Outlook 7:291–294, May 1959

———: Today's action will determine tomorrow's nursing. Nurs Outlook 13:38–41, September 1965

———: The significance of nursing care. Am J Nurs 61:63–66, November 1961

———: Theory in nursing: borrowed and unique. Nurs Res 17:206–209, May–June 1968

———: A philosophy of nursing. Nurs Outlook 7:198–200, April 1959

Johnson MM, Martin HW: A sociological analysis of the nurse role. Am J Nurs 58:373–377, March 1958

Johnson M: Pain—how do you know it's there and what do you do? Nurs '76 6:48–50, September 1976

Jordan JD: The nurse practitioner in a group practice. Am J Nurs 74:1447–1449, August 1974

Kelly KJ; An approach to the study of clinical inference in nursing. Nurs Res 13:314–322, fall 1964

———: Clinical inference in nursing—a nurse's viewpoint. Nurs Res 15:23–26, winter 1966

Kelly LY: The patient's right to know. Nurs Outlook 24:26–32, January 1976

———: Nursing practice acts. Am J Nurs 74:1310–1319, July 1974

Kelly NC: Nursing care plans. Nurs Outlook 14:61–64, May 1966

———: Needed: a comprehensive information system for nurses. Superv Nurse 2:38, May 1971

Kelly RL: Evaluation is more than measurement. Am J Nurs 73:114–116, January 1973

Ketefian S: Application of selected nursing research findings into nursing practice: a pilot study. Nurs Res 24:89–92, March–April 1975

King I: A conceptual frame of reference for nursing. Nurs Res 17:27–31, January–February 1968

King LS: What is a diagnosis? JAMA 202:154–157, November 20, 1967

Kinlein HL: Independent nurse practitioner. Nurs Outlook 20: 22–24, January 1972

Kinney AB, Blount M: Systems approach to myasthenia gravis. Nurs Clin N Am 6:435–453, September 1971

Kissinger JF, Ritzman RL, Seymour SF: Teaching medical-surgical nursing by concepts. Nurs Outlook 22:654–658, October 1974

Knight JH: Applying nursing process in the community. Nurs Outlook 22:708–711, November 1974

Knowles NL: Decision making in nursing—a necessity for doing. In: ANA Clinical Sessions, 1966. New York, Appleton-Century-Crofts, 1967

Komorita NI: Nursing Diagnosis, Am J Nurs 63:83–86, December 1963

Kraegel J, Schmidt V, Shukla RK, Goldsmith CE: A system of patient care based on patient needs. Nurs Outlook 20:257–264, April 1972

Kramer LA: The audit and I. Am J Nurs 76:1139–1141, July 1976

Kramer M: Concept formation. ANA 6th Nursing Research Conference, San Diego, California, April 8–10, 1970, pp 246–265

Kramer M: Nursing care plans-power to the patient. J Nurs Admin 2:29–34, September–October 1972

Kramer M, Egan E, Knauber J: The effect of presets on creative problem solving. Nurs Res 19:303–311, July–August 1970

Kreuter FR: What is good nursing care? Nurs Outlook 5:302–304, May 1957

La Belle B: Creative problem-solving techniques in nursing. J Creative Behavior 8(1):55–66, 1974

Lamberton MM: Primary health care–adult nurse clinician on a psychiatric unit. Am J Nurs 76:1961–1963, December 1976

Lambertsen EC: Nursing care plan should reflect present and future patient needs. Mod Hosp 103:128, October 1964

———: Nursing definition and philosophy precede nursing goal development. Mod Hosp 103:136, September 1964

———: Evaluating the quality of nursing care. Hospitals 39:61–66, November 1, 1965

Langford T: The evaluation of nursing: necessary and possible. Superv Nurse 2(11):65, 1971

Laverty F: Creative ideas through circumrelation. J Creative Behavior 8(1):40–46, 1974

Leininger NM: Nature of Science in nursing (introduction–conference on the nature of science in nursing). Nurs Res 18:388–389, September–October 1969

Levine ME: Adaptation and assessment: a rationale for nursing intervention. Am J Nurs 66:2450–2453, November 1966

———: The four conservation principles of nursing. Nurs Forum 6(1):45–59, 1967

———: The pursuit of wholeness. Am J Nurs 69:93–98, January 1969

Levinger G, Billings H: Nursing in a low-rent housing project. Am J Nurs 71:315–318, February 1971

Lewis GK: Communication: a factor in meeting emotional crises. Nurs Outlook 13:36–39, August 1965

Lewis L: This I believe . . . about the nursing process–key to care. Nurs Outlook 16:26–29, May 1968

Lewis MA: Child-initiated care. Am J Nurs 74:652–655, April 1974

Lindeman CA: Nursing Research: a visible, viable component of nursing practice. J Nurs Admin 3:18–21, March–April 1973

Little D, Carnevali D: The nursing care planning system. Nurs Outlook 19:164–167, March 1971

Lynaugh JE, Bates B: The two languages of nursing and medicine. Am J Nurs 73:66–69, January 1973

———: Physical diagnosis: a skill for all nurses? Am J Nurs 74:58–59, January 1974

MacGregor FC: Uncooperative patients: some cultural interpretations. Am J Nurs 67:88–91, January 1967

Malloy JL: Taking exception to problem-oriented nursing care. Am J Nurs 76:582–583, April 1976

Mansfield E: Care plans to stimulate learning. Am J Nurs 68: 2592–2593, December 1968

Manthey ME: A guide for interviewing. Am J Nurs 67:2088–2090, October 1967

Marshall J, Feeney S: Structured versus intuitive intake interview. Nurs Res 21:269–272, May–June 1972

Mathwig G: Nursing science. Image 3(1):9–14, 1969

———: Nursing science—the theoretical core of nursing knowledge. Image 4(1):20–23, 1971

Mauksch HO: It defies logic—but a hospital does function. Mod Hosp 95:67–70, October 1960

Mauksch IG, David ML: Prescription for survival. Am J Nurs 72: 2189–2193, December 1972

Mauksch IG, Young PR: Nurse-physician interaction in a family medical center. Nurs Outlook 22:113–119, February 1974

McCaffery M, Moss F: Nursing intervention for bodily pain. Am J Nurs 67:1224–1227, June 1967

McCain F: Nursing by assessment, not intuition. Am J Nurs 65: 82–84, April 1965

McCloskey JC: The nursing care plan: past, present, and uncertain future—a review of the literature. Nurs Forum 14(4): 364–382, 1975

———: The problem-oriented record vs the nursing care plan: a proposal. Nurs Outlook 23:492–495, August 1975

McClure M: Quality assurance and nursing education. A nursing service director's view. Nurs Outlook 24:367–369, June 1976

McDonald FJ, Harms MT: A theoretical model for an experimental curriculum. Nurs Outlook 14:48–51, August 1966

McGivern DO, Mezey MD, Baer ED: Teaching primary care in a baccalaureate program. Nurs Outlook 24:441–445, July 1976

McGriff EP: The courage for effective leadership in nursing. Image 8:56–60, October 1976

McGriff EP, Simms LL: Two New York nurses debate the NYSNA 1985 proposal. Am J Nurs 76:930–935, June 1976

McGuire RL: Bedside nursing audit. Am J Nurs 68:2146–2148, October 1968

McKay R: Theories, models, and systems for nursing. Nurs Res 18:393–399, September–October 1969

McPhetridge LM: Nursing history: one means to personalize care. Amer J Nurs 68:68–75, January 1968

———: Relationship of patients' responses to nursing history questions and selected factors: Preliminary study. Nurs Res 22:310–320, July–August 1973

Meleis AI: Role insufficiency and role supplementation: a conceptual framework. Nurs Res 24:264–271, July–August 1975

Meleis AI, Brenner P: Process or product evaluation? Nurs Outlook 23:303–307, May 1975

Mercadante LT: Leadership development seminars. Nurs Outlook, 13:59–61, September 1965

Merton R: The social nature of leadership. Am J Nurs 69:2614–2618, December 1969

Milio N: A broad perspective on health: a teaching-learning tool. Nurs Outlook 24:160–163, March 1976

Miller DI: Administration for the patient. Am J Nurs 65:114–116, July 1965

Miller J: Systems theory and family psychotherapy. Nurs Clin N Am 6:395–406, September, 1971

Minckley BB: Space and place in patient care. Am J Nurs 68:510–516, March 1968

Mitchell CE: Assessment of alcohol abuse. Nurs Outlook 24: 511–515, August 1976

Moritz DA, Sexton DL: Evaluation: a suggested method for appraising quality. J Nurs Educ 9(1):17, 1970

Moughton M: Systems and childhood psychosis. Nurs Clin N Am 6:425–434, September 1971

Mundinger MON, Jauron GD: Developing a nursing diagnosis. Nurs Outlook 23:94–98, February 1975

Munley MJ: An evaluation of nursing care by direct observation. Superv Nurse 4:28–34, April 1973

Murphy JF: Role expansion or role extension: some conceptual differences. Nurs Forum 9(4):380–390, 1970

Murray RLE: Caring. Am J Nurs 72:1286–1287, July 1972

Nadler G, Sahney V: A descriptive model of nursing care. Am J Nurs 69:336–341, February 1969

Naugle EH: Knock and wait. Am J Nurs 71:311–313, February 1971

———: The difference caring makes. Am J Nurs 73:1890–1891, November 1973

Nayer DD: The ANA position paper. Imprint, 23:23 ff, February 1976

Nehring V, Geach B: Patients' evaluation of their care: why they don't complain. Nurs Outlook 21:317–321, May 1973

Neshio K: Creative problem solving: a teaching innovation. Nurs Forum 6(4)432–441, 1967

Newman M: Identifying and meeting patients' needs in short-span nurse–patient relationships. Nurs Forum 5(1):76–86, 1966

———: Nursing's theoretical evolution. Nurs Outlook 20:450–453, July 1972

New York's "1985 Plan" goes to legislature; controversy over it deepens among nurses. Am J Nurs 76:878, June 1976

Nicholls M: Quality control in patient care. Am J Nurs 74:450–459, March 1974

Niland MB, Bentz PM: A problem-oriented approach to planning nursing care. Nurs Clin N Am 9:235–245, June 1974

Norris C: Toward a science of nursing. Nurs Forum 3(3):10–45, 1964

———: Delusions that trap nurses. Nurs Outlook 21:18–21, January 1973

Nursing is coming of age—through the practitioner movement. Pro-Mauksch IG, Con-Rogers ME. Am J Nurs 75:1834–1843, October 1975

Oelbaum CH: Hallmarks of adult wellness. Am J Nurs 74:1623–1625, September 1974

Orem D: The hope of nursing. J Nurs Educ 1(1):5–7, January 1962

Orme JY, Lindbeck RS: Nurse participation in medical peer review. Nurs Outlook 22:27–30, January 1974

O'Shea HS: A guide to evaluation of clinical performance. Am J Nurs 67:1877–1879, September 1967

Palmer J: Management by objectives. J Nurs Administr 1:17–23, January–February 1971

Pankratz D, Pankratz L: The nursing care plan: theory and reality. Superv Nurse 4:51–55, April 1973

Pardee G, Hoshaw DO, Huber CJ, Larson BA: Patient care evaluation is every nurses' job. Am J Nurs 71:1958–1960, October 1971

Parker W: Medication histories. Am J Nurs 76:1969–1971, December 1976

Parnes SJ: Creativity: developing human potential. J Creative Behavior 5(1):19–36, 1971

Parsons MC, Stephens G: Postoperative complications: assessment and intervention. Am J Nurs 74:240–244, February 1974

Patterson EA, Stence FL: Thinking together to solve care problems. Am J Nurs 70:1703–1706, August 1970

Peabody SR: Assessment and planning for continuity of care from hospital to home. Nurs Clin N Am 4:303–310, June 1969

Perrine G: Needs met and unmet. Am J Nurs 71:2128–2133, November 1971

Perry JH: Written nursing care plans. Hosp Prog 71–73, July 1963

Peterson CJ, Hass RC, Killalea MA: Theoretical framework for an associate degree curriculum. Nurs Outlook 22:321–324, May 1974

Peterson GG: What head nurses look for when evaluating assignments. Am J Nurs 73:641–644, April 1973

Peterson LW: Operant approach to observation and recording. Nurs Outlook 15:28–32, 1967

Petrlik JC: Diabetic peripheral neuropathy. Am J Nurs 76: 1794–1797, November 1976

Pfaudler M: After stroke. Am J Nurs 73:1892–1896, November 1973

Phaneuf MC: Quality assurance: a nursing view. Hospitals 47:62 ff, October 16, 1973

———: A nursing audit method. Nurs Outlook 12:42–45, May 1964

———: The nursing audit for evaluation of patient care. Nurs Outlook 14:51–54, June 1966

Pluckhan ML: Space: The silent language. Nurs Forum 7(4):386–397, 1968

Poland M, English N, Thornton N, Owens D: PETO—A system for assessing and meeting patient care needs. Am J Nurs 70:1479–1482, July 1970

Pollok C, Poteet G, Whelan W: Students' rights. Am J Nurs 76: 600–703, April 1976

Preston T: When words fail. Am J Nurs 73:2064–2066, December 1973

Price E: Data processing, present and potential. Am J Nurs 67: 2558–2564, December 1967

Quinn N, Somers AR: The patients' bill of rights: a significant aspect of the consumer revolution. Nurs Outlook 24:243, April 1974

Ramey IG: Setting nursing standards and evaluating care. J Nurs Admin 3(9):27, 1973

Ramphal M: The patient is the center of nursing. Maryland Nurs News spring:13–20, 1968

———: Peer review. Am J Nurs 74:63–67, January 1974

Reilly DE: Why a conceptual framework? Nurs Outlook 23:566–569, September 1975

Reiter F: The nurse clinician. Am J Nurs 66:274–280, February 1966

———: Choosing the better part. Am J. Nurs 64:65–68, December 1964

Reres M: Systems analysis: an approach to working with personality disorders. Nurs Clin N Am 6:455–462, September 1971

Rinaldi LA, Rubin CF: Adding retrospective audit. Am J Nurs 75:256–259, February 1975

Rinaldi LA, Kelly B: What to do after the audit is done. Am J Nurs 77:268–269, February 1977

Roach LB: Assessing changes in dark skin. Nurs '72 2:19–22, November 1972

———: Assessing skin changes—the subtle and the obvious. Nurs '74 3:64–67, March 1974

———: Assessment—color changes in dark skin. Nurs '77 7:48–51, January 1977

Roberts SL: Skin assessment for color and temperature. Am J Nurs 75:610–613, April 1975

Rogers M: Euphemisms in nursing's future. Image 7(2):3–9, 1975

Rosen A, Abraham GE: Evaluation of a procedure for assessing the performance of staff nurses. Nurs Res 12:78–82, spring 1963

Rosen A. Performance appraisal interviewing evaluated by professional observers. Nurs Res 16:32–37, winter 1967

Rothberg JS: Why nursing diagnosis? Am J Nurs 67:1040–1042, May 1967

Rothwell MG: A patient-centered group practice. Nurs Outlook 24:745–748, December 1976

Routhier R: Tools for the evaluation of patient care. Superv Nurse 3(1):15, January 1972

Roy C: Adaptation: a conceptual framework for nursing. Nurs Outlook 18:42–45, March 1970

———: Adaptation: a basis for nursing practice. Nurs Outlook 19:254–257, April 1971

———: Adaptation: implications for curriculum change. Nurs Outlook 21:163–168, March 1973

———: A diagnostic classification system for nursing. Nurs Outlook 23:90–94, February 1975

Roznoy MS: The young adult-taking a sexual history. Am J Nurs 76:1279–1282, August 1976

Rubin CF, et al: Nursing audit-nurses evaluating nursing. Am J Nurs 72:916–921, May 1972

———: Auditing the decubitus ulcer problem. Am J Nurs 74: 1820–1821, October 1974

Rubin R: A theory of clinical nursing. Nurs Res 17:210–212, May–June, 1968

Ruby E: Early omens of cerebral disaster. Nurs '77 7:58–62, February 1977

Rushing W: The hospital nurse as a mother surrogate and bedside psychologist. Ment Hyg 50:71–79, 1966

Ruybal SE, Bauwens E, Fasla M: Community assessment: an epidemiological approach, Nurs Outlook 23:365–368, June 1975

Ryan BJ: Nursing care plans: a systems approach to developing criteria for planning and evaluation. J Nurs Admin 3:50–57, May–June 1973

Ryan R: Thrombophlebitis: assessment and prevention. Am J Nurs 76:1634–1636, October 1976

Sanazaro PJ, Slosberg B: Patient care evaluation. Hospitals 40(7): 131, 1971

Schaefer J: The inter-relatedness of decision making and the nursing process. Am J Nurs 74:1852–1855, October 1974

Schaefer MJ: How should we organize? J Nurs Admin 6:13, February 1976

Schell PL, Campbell AT: Problem-oriented medical records. POMR —not just another way to chart. Nurs Outlook 20:510–514, August 1972

Schimpf K: The human body as an energy system. Am J Nurs 71:117–120, January 1971

Schmidt J: Availability: a concept of nursing practice. Am J Nurs 72:1086–1089, June 1972

Schueler A: Utilization review for medicare—does it open a new gap in services? Am J Nurs 77:110–111, January 1977

Scuffle P: Report of the task force to study the implications of the recommendations presented in *An Abstract for Action*. Nurs Outlook 21:111–118, February 1973

Shelter MG: Operating room nurses go visiting. Am J Nurs 72: 1266–1269, July 1972

Shields M: A model apt for measurement. Nurs Outlook 19:600–601, September 1971

Simmons HE, Ball JR: PSRO and the dissolution of the malpractice suit. Book excerpt in J Fam Practice 4(2):244–261, 1977

Smith DM: A clinical nursing tool. Am J Nurs 68:2384–2388, November 1968

———: Writing objectives as a nursing practice skill. Am J Nurs 71:319–320, February 1971

Snider ME: Utilization review for medicare–is this a good use of nurses' time? Am J Nurs 77:107–109, January 1977

Snyder JC, Wilson FM: Elements of a psychological assessment, Am J Nurs 77:235–239, February 1977

Snyder M, Baum R: Assessing Station and Gait. Am J Nurs 74: 1256–1257, July 1974

Sprathen LP: Evaluating mental health status with a simplified rating scale. J Psych Nurs and Mental Health Serv 11(5):37–41, September–October 1973

Standeven M: The relevant who of problem solving. Nurs Forum 10(2):166–175, 1971

Statement on diploma nurse education. The Am Nurse 5:June 1973

Stetler CB, Marram G: Evaluating research findings for applicability in practice. Nurs Outlook 24:559–563, September 1976

Stevens BJ: Why won't nurses write nursing care plans? J Nurs Admin 2(6):6, 1972

Strauss A, Fagerhaugh SY, Glaser B: Pain: an organizational-work-interactional perspective. Nurs Outlook 22:560–566, September 1974

Study of credentialing launched. Am J Nurs 76:1893–1895, December 1976

Styles MM: In the name of integration. Nurs Outlook 24:738–744, December 1976

Schwartz DR: Toward more precise evaluation of patients' needs. Nurs Outlook 13:42–44, May 1965

Symposium on a systems approach to nursing. Nurs Clin N Am 6:383–462, September 1971

Talabere L, Graves P: A tool for assessing families of burned children. Am J Nurs 76:225–227, February 1976

Tapia JA: The nursing process in family health. Nurs Outlook 20:267–270, April 1972

Taylor JW: Measuring the outcomes of nursing care. Nurs Clin N Am 9:337–348, June 1974

Taylor SD: Bibliography on nursing research, 1950–1974. Nurs Res 24:207–225, May–June 1975

Theis C, Harrington H: Three factors that affect practice–communications, assignments, attitudes. Am J Nurs 68:1478–1482, July 1968

Thigpen LW, Drane JW: The Venn diagram: a tool for conceptualization in nursing. Nurs Res 16:252–260, summer 1967

Thom AM, Stafford K: Time for evaluation of services. Hospitals 46(19):57, 1972

Thoma D, Pittman K: Evaluation of problem-oriented nursing notes. J Nurs Admin 2(3):50–52, May–June 1972

Thomas LA: Predicting change in nursing values. J Nurs Admin 1(3):50, 1971

Travelbee J: To find meaning in illness. Nurs '72 2:6–8, December 1972

Traver GA: Assessment of thorax and lungs. Am J Nurs 73:466–471, March 1973

Turnbull SJ: Shifting the focus to health. Am J Nurs 76:1985–1987, December 1976

Vaillot MC: Existentialism: a philosophy of commitment. Am J Nurs 66:500–505, March 1966

———: Nursing theory, levels of nursing, and curriculum development. Nurs Forum 9(3):234–249, 1970

Vincent P: Some crucial terms in nursing–a second opinion. Nurs Outlook 23:46–48, January 1975

Wagner B: Care plans: right, reasonable, and reachable. Am J Nurs 69:986–990, May 1969

Wagner P: Testing the Roy adaptation model in practice. Nurs Outlook 24:682–685, November 1976

Wald FS, Leonard RC: Towards development of nursing practice theory, Nurs Res 13:309–313, fall 1964

Walker LO: Toward a clearer understanding of the concept of nursing theory. Nurs Res 20:428–435, September–October 1971

Walker V, McReynolds D, Patrick E: A care plan for ailing nurses' notes. Am J Nurs 65:74–76, August 1965

Webb KJ: Early assessment of orthopedic injuries. Am J Nurs 74:1048–1052, June 1974

Weed LL: Medical records that guide and teach. New Engl J Med 278:598–599, 652–657, March 14, 21, 1968

Whiting JF: Patient's needs, nurse's needs and the healing process. Am J Nurs 59:661–665, May 1959

Wiedenbach E: The helping art of nursing. Am J Nurs 63:54–57, November 1963

———: Comment on: "Beliefs and values: Bases for curriculum design," Nurs Res 17:427, September–October 1970

Wiener CL: Pain Assessment on an orthopedic ward. Nurs Outlook 23:508–516, August 1975

Willacker J: Bowel sounds. Am J Nurs 73:2100–2101, December 1973

Williams DH: Sleep and disease. Am J Nurs 71:2321–2334, December 1971

Wilson R: PSRO's in nursing: what are they? Imprint 23:36–37, April 1976

Winslow EH, Fuhs FM: Preoperative assessment for postoperative evaluation. Am J Nurs 73:1372–1374, August 1973

Wolff IS: Acceptance. Am J Nurs 72:1412–1415, August 1972

Wolff H, Erickson R: The assessment man. Nurs Outlook 25: 103–107, February 1977

Wood V: Measurement and evaluation in nursing education. Can Nurse 62:54–58, April 1966

Woods MF: Measuring a patient's needs and progress. Nurs Outlook 14:38–41, October 1966

Woody M, Mallison M: The problem-oriented system for patient centered care. Am J Nurs 73:1168–1175, July 1973

Yarnall SR, Atwood J: Problem-oriented practice for nurses and physicians. Nurs Clin N Am 9:215–218, June 1974

Young R (ed.), Quality patient care. Can Nurse 61:975–78, December 1965

Yura H: Nursing leadership behavior. Superv Nurs 2:55–64, February 1971

Zderad L: Empathetic nursing. Nurs Clin N Am 4:655–662, December 1969

Zimmer MJ: Quality assurance for outcomes of patient care. Nurs Clin N Am 9:305–315, June 1974

Zimmerman DS, Gohrke C: The goal-directed nursing approach: it does work. Am J Nurs 70:306–310, February 1970

Unpublished

Crenshaw AE: Invasion of Personal Space as Perceived by a Selected Group of Patients. Unpublished Masters Dissertation, School of Nursing, The Catholic University of America, Washington, DC, May 1972

Gangwer ME: Identification of Crucial Information for a Nursing

History. Unpublished Masters Dissertation, Washington, DC, The Catholic University of America, School of Nursing, 1965

Gordon M: Strategies in Probabilistic Concept Attainment: A Study of Nursing Diagnosis. Boston, Mass., Boston College, 1972 (Doctoral Dissertation)

Horgan MV: Concepts about Nursing in Selected Nursing Literature from 1950–1965. Unpublished Masters Dissertation, Washington, DC, The Catholic University of America, School of Nursing, 1967

Lusted LB, Stahl WR: Conceptual Models of Diagnosis. In: Jacquez, John A (ed): The Diagnostic Process. Ann Arbor, University of Michigan, 1964 (mimeographed)

McMullan D: A Study to Formulate Principles of Nursing Pertaining to Nursing Diagnosis and Nursing Therapy Which Underlie Professional Nursing Practice. New York, New York University, 1962 (Doctoral Dissertation)

Films

The Pulses Profile. New York State Department of Health, 1970, 16 mm; Amer J Nurs Film Library, c/o Association-Sterling Films, 600 Grand Avenue, Ridgefield, N.J. 07657

Programmed Instruction

Programmed Instruction Series: Patient Assessment, New York, Am J Nurs

Taking a Patient's History	February 1974	pp. 293–324
Examination of the Abdomen	September 1974	pp. 1679–1702
Examination of the Eye, Part I	November 1974	pp. 2039–2062
Examination of the Eye, Part II	January 1975	pp. 105–128
Examination of the Ear,	March 1975	pp. 459–475
Examination of the Head and Neck	May 1975	pp. 839–862
Neurological Examination, Part I	September 1975	pp. 1511–1536
Neurological Examination, Part II	November 1975	pp. 2037–2062
Neurological Examination, Part III	April 1976	pp. 609–633
Blood Gas and Acid–Base Concepts in Respiratory Care,	June 1976	pp. 963–992
Examination of the Chest and Lungs	September 1976	pp. 1453–1475
Examination of the Heart and Great Vessels, Part I	November 1976	pp. 1807–1830
Auscultation of the Heart, Part II	February 1977	pp. 275–298

Index

Notes